KU-603-951

The Health Services of Ireland

Do Mháire, mo bhean chéile

NWHB Ballybofey Library

The Health Services of Ireland

Brendan Hensey
D.Econ.Sc., D.P.A. (N.U.I.)

Institute of Public Administration
Dublin

© 1959, 1972, 1979 Institute of Public
Administration

ISBN O 902173 86 3

All rights reserved. No part of
this publication may be reproduced
or transmitted in any form or by
any means, electronic or mechanical,
including photocopy, recording,
or any information storage and
retrieval system, without permission
in writing from the publisher.

Published by
Institute of Public Administration
59 Lansdowne Road
Dublin 4
Ireland

First Published 1959
Second Edition 1972
Third Edition 1979

Set in 12pt. Plantin and printed
by Iona Print Ltd., Dublin

CONTENTS

Note to Third Edition

Twenty years a-growing—as have been our health services, so has *The Health Services of Ireland*. The book has increased in size mainly because this edition includes further appendixes on the details of the services. I hope these will be found useful to those using the work as a handbook for administration, while not distracting students of the system as a whole.

Once more I must thank those in the Department—too many to mention them all —who have helped in the revisions needed for this edition. As in the case of the second edition, Tadgh Tansley acted with great energy and efficiency as research assistant and general co-ordinator of the revisions and additions to the text and I am particularly indebted to him. I would also like to express my appreciation of the work done so skillfully by Tony Farmar of the Institute of Public Administration in the editing of the text of this edition and in its production.

BRENDAN HENSEY

May, 1979

Chapter One

The Growth of the Health Services—The Nineteenth Century

'Health services' may be defined as those services under which public authorities arrange for the diagnosis, prevention and treatment of human illness. The purpose of this book is to explain what the health services are, how they originated, how they are operated, who is entitled to them and how much they cost. It is concerned with the relationships of the State and public bodies with, on the one hand, the medical profession and its ancillaries and, on the other hand, the general public. These relationships have developed from the increasing recognition of the fact that simple private arrangements between practitioners as individuals and patients could not offer to the general public the full benefits of an expanding medical science. Some form of organisation of health services became essential once discoveries in that science began to move out of the fields of homely palliatives and simple empirical cures. This factor did not, of course, determine the exact form of the organisation which has developed. That is a complex function of sociology and economics.

One cannot pick a single point of time and say that the modern trend towards the development of health services commenced then. The source of a broad river is often a number of insignificant rivulets which only become noticeable when they combine to form the main stream or a substantial tributary. Such rivulets leading to the stream of the developing health services can, by painstaking search, be discerned from an early period but it is only in the latter part of the eighteenth and the early part of the nineteenth century that they have joined to become a steady flow.

No clear-cut social policy could be said to have influenced the establishment of such services as were brought into existence in the eighteenth century. The latter half of that century saw the commencement of the local authority hospital system with the establishment of county infirmaries and fever hospitals under the management of committees on which the public authorities were represented. The mental treatment ser-

1

vice originated in the same period and developed early in the nineteenth century, when the Grand Juries had power to raise funds towards the support of lunatic asylums and legislation was passed delimiting the districts for mental hospital services. The year 1818 saw the first provision for the appointment of local boards of health to organise preventive services. History does not record that these boards were very successful in achieving their objective.

The provision of these services, such as they were, was rather in contradiction to the laissez-faire economic and social policies prevalent at the time. Each of the services was designed to meet a demand which could not be answered by referring to the current social theory. Sick paupers had to be housed, fevers could not be left to spread unchecked and lunatics had to be confined. It was these hard facts, and not any clear vision of where they were moving, that influenced public representatives and administrators to attempt what was done at the time.

The acceptance of Benthamite philosophy in the first half of the nineteenth century as a basis for the social policies of the then United Kingdom of Great Britain and Ireland introduced a more positive influence in the development of health services. To revert to our riverine metaphor, two strong streams from this source developed at the time, to diverge and meet later on the broad plains of the twentieth century. The first of these streams moved through the dismal countryside of the Poor Law; the second was channelled in a business-like fashion by the medical officers and engineers in charge of environmental sanitation.

The story of the development of the health services from the early nineteenth century to the present day falls into two parts—the establishment of the organs of administration and the introduction and improvement of the services themselves. We propose to relate these two parts of the story, first for the period up to the end of the nineteenth century and in later chapters for the twentieth century.

Administration

Central administration
In the early nineteenth century there was no central authority

established specially for the administration of health services. Such functions as fell to be discharged at the centre in relation to the lunatic asylums and the other services which existed then were discharged by the Lord Lieutenant or his subordinates. The year 1838 saw the first departure from this. The Poor Law Act of that year established a tightly-organised administration for the relief of the poor, which became responsible for the development of a number of the health services. Substantial powers were reserved under this legislation to the central authority, which in the first instance was the English Poor Law Commissioners. While this body accomplished its initial task of equipping the country with workhouses,[1] the remoteness of the Commissioners from the work in Ireland made the arrangement an unsatisfactory one for the continued operation of the services. In 1847, the Irish Poor Law Commissioners were appointed to take over the functions of the English Commissioners.[2]

The Irish Poor Law Commissioners were appointed by the Queen. Their task was to ensure uniformity in the poor law services and they exercised very detailed control over the local authorities providing them. Their field of action was, however, limited to the poor law services. Other local government services (and in particular the sanitary services) were developing at the time and the need for a central co-ordinating authority grew. The Royal Sanitary Commission of 1869 reported in favour of a Government-appointed board to take over the functions of the Poor Law Commissioners and be responsible also for the supervising of the other services. The Irish Local Government Board was, in accordance with this recommendation, established in 1872[3] and remained the central authority for the local government and health services until the third decade of the twentieth century.

The Irish Local Government Board consisted of five members, under the presidency of the Chief Secretary to the Lord Lieutenant. One of the members was required to be medically qualified. The Board exercised only the executive

---

[1]An account of the building of the workhouses is given in an article by P. J. Meghen in *Administration* Vol. 3, No. 1 Spring 1955.
[2]See the Poor Relief (Ireland) Act, 1847.
[3]Under the Irish Local Government Board Act, 1872.

functions of a central authority. Its duty was to administer
policy as laid down in the Acts of Parliament and it was no part
of the Board's work to sponsor legislation as a Minister of State
does. Most of the services which will be subsequently described
fell within the Board's province of administration, but an important exclusion from that province was the mental treatment
service, which remained apart under the Lord Lieutenant. The
Inspector of Mental Hospitals, one of his officers, had considerable autonomous powers in the supervision of this service.

Local Administration
Local health service administration developed within the local
government system, for which the nineteenth century was a
period of considerable change and development. The trend was
towards greater uniformity in the pattern of authorities and a
widening of the franchise on which they were elected. Each of
the classes of authorities then established and developed was
responsible for a number of local services but, in the allocation
of these, the health services were not viewed as a unit. There
was no apparent endeavour to rationalise and co-ordinate at a
local level the administration of the health services then
developing. Generally speaking, each service, as it was introduced, was made the responsibility of whichever of the existing set of local authorities was considered to be the most convenient. In stating this, a reservation should be made for the
mental treatment service. The maintenance and financing of
lunatic asylums remained the responsibility of committees of
management specially appointed for the purpose by the central
authority. These committees were not truly local authorities in
the present day meaning of the term, but they were at the time
the only group of bodies specially created for the provision of a
health service.

Two main sets of local authorities became concerned during
this period with the provision of the services—the boards of
guardians and the sanitary authorities. The boards of guardians were the local agents of the Poor Law Commissioners,
having come into being under the Act of 1838 referred to
earlier. They were bodies with membership made up of justices
of the peace and persons elected by the ratepayers. Each of
these authorities served a district known as the Poor Law

Union, there being one hundred and twenty-six of these in the present area of the State.

The Poor Law administration had been primarily set up to provide physical necessities for paupers. Its role in the health services was at first not significant but, during the decades up to 1900, this role grew in importance.

In the meantime, the sanitary authorities were evolving. These were to play an important part in developing the preventive side of the health services. There were sanitary authorities in towns since the early nineteenth century, their work consisting mainly of the provision of sewers, water-supplies, wash-houses, street lighting and other amenities conducive to comfort and health. Personal health services were at first no important part of their functions and it was not until the sanitary administration was re-organised under the Public Health (Ireland) Acts of 1874 and 1878 that this side of their work assumed prominence. Under those Acts, the existing municipal corporations and town commissioners were appointed as sanitary authorities for the larger urban areas. No special rural sanitary authorities were constituted then; the boards of guardians became the sanitary authorities for the rural areas and smaller towns.

The final change in the nineteenth century administration came with the Local Government (Ireland) Act, 1898. Under that Act there were established elective county councils, urban district councils and rural district councils. The last-mentioned councils were appointed for the rural sanitary districts and took over the sanitary functions of the boards of guardians. The latter remained, however, to discharge their original functions of providing relief (including medical relief) for the poor. The county councils took over the administration (either direct or through joint committees) of the district lunatic asylums but were not otherwise concerned at the time with the health services.

Finance
The primary source of money for the health services which were then developed was local taxation. Some State aid was provided towards the end of the century from the Estate Duty Grant and the Licence Duty Grant. The Estate Duty Grant

was introduced in 1888.[4] The total grant each year was calculated as being a sum equivalent to one and one-half per cent of the net value of the property in respect of which Estate Duty was leviable each year. The grant was paid for a number of local services, including those of the Poor Law authorities. The Licence Duty Grant, which was introduced in 1898,[5] was designed to recoup specified proportions of the cost of particular items in the services. The Grant was intended to meet the following:

(a) one-half of the salaries of the medical officers of workhouses and dispensaries;

(b) one-half of the salary of one trained nurse in each workhouse, who was actually employed and possessed the prescribed qualifications;

(c) the whole of the salaries of schoolmasters and schoolmistresses in the workhouses;

(d) one-half of the cost of medicines and medical and surgical appliances;

(e) one-half of the salaries of officers of sanitary authorities;

(f) a capitation grant for inmates of lunatic asylums at a rate not exceeding four shillings a week.

The relative importance attached to financial incentives for the development in the workhouses of medical and nursing services on the one hand and schooling on the other hand, will be noticed. The funds for this Grant were derived from fees for certain local licences. If the total of these was insufficient to meet the commitments, the grant for each purpose was abated proportionately—a procedure which called for no mean volume of calculations.

These grants had what was an advantage to the Treasury and a disadvantage to the health administration in that they were related to the yield of specified taxes. They could not be used as an incentive to the local authorities for the general development of the services as the amount available was not sufficient to meet more than a small proportion of the cost. We

---

[4]The Grant, which was originally the Probate Duty Grant, was first established under the Probate Duties (Ireland) Act, 1888. The name was changed to the Estate Duty Grant by the Finance Act, 1894.

[5]By section 58 of the Local Government (Ireland) Act, 1898.

shall see how these grants were absorbed in 1947 into a more rational and generous system of State aid towards local health expenditure.

The nineteenth century services

General hospitals and workhouses
By the early nineteenth century several voluntary hospitals had been developed, mostly in Dublin. Infirmaries had also been provided in a number of areas under special local Acts. Outside the areas served by the voluntary hospitals, there was, however, nothing in the nature of a general hospital system. Such a system was developed from the year 1838 on, not at first as a result of a deliberate policy to provide for the rest of the country the same type of services as the voluntary hospitals provided in Dublin, but as an adjunct to a service for the maintenance of the ablebodied destitute in institutions.

The primary duty of the boards of guardians—to maintain poor persons 'unable by their own industry or other lawful means' to provide for themselves—was discharged in the workhouses erected by the Poor Law Commissioners. The workhouses were designed to be grim and strictly functional—deliberately so, as it was a tenet of the Poor Law to discourage all but the absolutely destitute from its benefits. They could not be described as hospitals in the present-day meaning of the term but, as time went by, hospital services were developed in them.

We shall see how in the twentieth century the poor law administration became responsible for the greater part of the general hospital system outside Dublin. In the nineteenth century, however, what was done by the boards of guardians by way of providing hospital services in the workhouses was limited, not only by the restricted outlook of the authorities on their duty towards the sick poor, but also because medical science had not yet developed to the stage where the hospital services could provide the benefits they do to-day.

Mental health
The care of the mentally ill formed perhaps the greatest single unit in the health services of the time. Institutions were

provided throughout the entire country but, of course, they were simply lunatic asylums. Proper treatment and nursing of the mentally ill was a matter for the future.

The dispensary service
The dispensary service is generally regarded as having been initiated in the year 1851, when the Act known as the Medical Charities Act was passed.[6] This Act consolidated a dispensary service which had been developing in several areas. It placed on the Poor Law Commissioners the duty of seeing that the boards of guardians provided dispensaries and appointed medical officers. Each Poor Law Union was divided into a number of dispensary districts, which remained the basic areas of health administration until 1970. The dispensary doctor was given the duty of attending, without charge, to the sick poor in his district who were identified through the issue of 'red tickets' by authorised persons in the Poor Law system. He was entitled to attend to those outside this class as a private practitioner. The development of the dispensary system led to the country being served uniformly at the general practitioner level.

Registration of births, deaths and marriages
The development of the dispensary system facilitated the introduction of the civil registration of births and deaths and the extension of the system for the registration of marriages. In 1863, the dispensary doctors were made registrars of births and deaths and of Catholic marriages (other marriages were registered under a different earlier system).[7] The dispensary doctor, in his capacity of registrar, was subject to a Superintendent Registrar, who was usually the Clerk of the Poor Law Union. The entire system was made subject to the Registrar General, an autonomous official appointed by the Lord Lieutenant. This important side-line of the Poor Law services was to be the source in later years of many of the vital statistics which formed the basis of plans for further development in the health services.

Preventive services
The periodic occurrence of epidemics of the pestilences which

---

[6]The proper title of the Act is the Poor Relief (Ireland) Act, 1851.
[7]See Chapter 13.

were common in Ireland in the nineteenth century spurred the Government to spasmodic efforts to control them and alleviate their effects. Temporary commissioners of health were, for example, appointed at the time of the Great Famine and these acted in some respects through the local boards of guardians. Anything done at this time was unsystematic and, with the exception of smallpox vaccination, which was introduced in 1858, none of the measures of that time could be regarded as a forerunner of our present preventive services. It was not until the work of Chadwick, Simon and others in Britain punched home the connection between environment and infectious diseases and led to the introduction there of a systemised effective sanitary law, that serious attention was given to the development of the sanitary services and the preventive health services in Ireland.

Sanitary services could not realistically be organised except by public authorities; neither could the preventive services which were their ancillary. Thus, at a time when curative medicine, inside and outside hospitals, was still largely left to individuals and private organisations, the preventive services became a clear-cut responsibility of the public authorities. The earlier piecemeal efforts were drawn together and codified in the Public Health (Ireland) Act, 1878. This was closely modelled on an earlier English Act and was designed mainly to give a single body of law on the provision of water supplies, sewerage works and similar services. The provisions of the Act relating to the health services, as we have defined them, comprise only a small part of the whole code but they were until 1947 the legal basis for a considerable sector of the health services.

The most important provisions in the Act from our point of view were those under which power was given to the Local Government Board to make regulations to prevent the spread of infectious diseases. Food hygiene controls also originated in this Act, which contained prohibitions on the sale of food which was 'diseased, contaminated, or otherwise unfit for human consumption.' The dispensary doctors under this Act became holders of a separate and additional office of medical officer of health, with duties related mainly to the control of infectious diseases. In the cities of Dublin, Cork, Limerick and Waterford, medical superintendent officers of health were appointed to supervise and co-ordinate the work of the local medical officers of health, but in the rural areas the co-ordination and supervision of the work of the district medical officers of health remained entirely with the medical inspectors of the Local Government Board.

The position at the end of the century

The nineteenth century had seen the evolution of three sets of authorities to administer respectively the mental health services, the Poor Law services and the preventive services. None of these was equipped or encouraged to consider the health services as a whole. Centrally, the Local Government Board had the appearance of an authority which could co-ordinate the development of the services. It must be remembered, however, that the Board's functions were limited, firstly by its not being concerned with the lunatic asylums and secondly by its not being responsible for the evolution of policy in Parliament. Furthermore, the dichotomy between the Poor Law and the law on the preventive services appears to have hindered the development within the Board of a unified outlook on the services.

The services provided and developed under this administration were mixed in quality. The dispensary medical service was regarded as performing its function well but, on the other hand, the workhouse system was never viewed with any feeling warmer than toleration. The hospital service associated with it was no more popular. The preventive services had had some important successes—notably in the virtual elimination of smallpox and typhus—and were confidently looking forward to the conquest of other infectious diseases.

As a whole, however, the practical results achieved in improving the general standard of health were not noteworthy. The death-rate, at 17·7 per 1,000 population at the turn of the century, had not varied to any extent since it was first calculated in the eighteen-sixties and the infant mortality rate had actually increased from 95·7 per 1,000 live births in the eighteen-sixties to 99·4 in the eighteen-nineties. It would, however, be as unreasonable to blame this lack of progress entirely on the deficiencies in the scope and organisation of the health services of the day, as it would be to give the entire credit for the spectacular improvements in the twentieth century to the development in that century of health services as such. Medical science in the nineteenth century was not so developed that better organisation of services could have achieved a great deal.

Chapter Two

The period 1900 to 1945

The story of the services in the twentieth century falls naturally into two parts, that for the period up to the end of the Second World War and the account of the developments since then. The first of these periods was one in which the scope and tempo of the changes made were relatively narrow and slow.

Administration

Central administration
No change was made by the United Kingdom government in central administration and the changes which did come in this period were incidental to the War of Independence and the achievement of self-government. During that war the British authorities had maintained the Local Government Board in Dublin as the central authority, but a department of local government set up by Dáil Éireann was increasingly recognised by the local councils. For a while, therefore, there were two central authorities but, with the political settlement of the early twenties, the Local Government Board ceased to exist. Under the Ministers and Secretaries Act, 1924, the Department of Local Government and Public Health, under its own minister, became the statutory central authority for the services and took over the administration of the law previously the responsibility of the Local Government Board. The Custom House in Dublin, which, as the headquarters of the Board, was burned with most of its records during the War of Independence, was rebuilt and again became the centre of local government and health administration.

There were two important differences between the new central authority and the Board it replaced. Firstly, it was in the charge of a Minister of State who was no mere administrator of policy but a member of the Government specially designated as the prime mover in the making of policy and the

12

preparation and introduction of new health legislation. Secondly, it was responsible for all the health services, because the Minister for Local Government and Public Health took over also the Lord Lieutenant's duties in relation to the lunatic asylums.

Local administration
No important changes were made in local administration before the War of Independence, the most noteworthy development of the period being that the county councils were given functions in relation to the tuberculosis and school medical services when they were initiated. These councils were undoubtedly the most suitable of the existing sets of authorities for those services, but their introduction into the field of general health services added one more set of authorities to the boards of guardians and sanitary authorities who already had responsibilities in that field.

The achievement of self-government brought with it a number of far-reaching changes in the local administration of the claims for other benefits of the National Health Insurance the less beneficent side of the former administration, were abolished and were replaced by county boards of assistance. This change was initiated under rather informal 'county schemes' which subsequently received the sanction of Parliament in the Local Government (Temporary Provisions) Act, 1923. The rural district councils were abolished in 1925[1] and, except in a few areas, their sanitary functions were taken over by the bodies which had replaced the boards of guardians. These bodies then became boards of health and public assistance. They were appointed by the county councils and the membership of each was made up of ten members of the parent council. The new bodies were responsible for the Poor Law services for the entire county, but were in charge of the sanitary and preventive health services only in the rural districts. The urban district councils and their functions as sanitary authorities were not affected by the change. Neither were the county councils, which retained responsibility for the mental health service, the tuberculosis service and the school medical service.

[1]Under the Local Government Act, 1925.

Check this page with Leo

Nothing much by way of simplification was effected by these changes, the main practical achievement being the elimination of the smaller rural local authorities (the boards of guardians and the rural district councils). However, the Act which consolidated the new local administration also provided for the appointment of county medical officers of health. This office was analogous to that of the medical superintendent officers of health who were provided for the county boroughs in 1878. The county medical officer of health was an officer of the county council and was made responsible for the efficient operation of the tuberculosis service and the school medical service administered by the council. He was, however, also responsible for the infectious diseases services, the maternity and child welfare services and the other preventive services which were the responsibility of the boards of health and public assistance in rural areas and of the urban district councils in the urban districts. Through the county medical officer of health, co-ordination could be effected among these services, but it must be remembered that his responsibilities did not extend to the dispensary medical service, the general hospital service or the treatment of mental diseases.

These arrangements for local administration lasted until the early years of the Second World War, when they were substantially altered by the introduction of the county management system. The management system, under which one officer took over responsibility for the day-to-day executive functions of the elected members of a local body, had been introduced earlier for the Corporations of Dublin, Cork, Limerick and Waterford. By the County Management Act, 1940, it was extended to all areas. As a corollary to this step, the boards of health and public assistance (which were, to a large extent, merely executive committees of the county councils) were abolished, their work being taken over by the county councils and the managers. The urban district councils remained, but the county manager acted for them as well as for the county council.

The significance of these changes lay in the fact that the county managers took over all the detailed administrative work and much of the formulation of local policy on all the health services. However, the law still recognised the distinction between public assistance authorities, sanitary authorities and mental hospital authorities, and the three divisions of the services were not at this point integrated to any significant extent. Nevertheless, the alterations made by the introduction of county management set the stage for some fundamental rethinking after the war on several aspects of the services and their administration.

Finance
The basis for financing the services remained unchanged during this period. The local rates continued to meet most of the cost, but for some services rather more generous state assistance was provided. Special grants were introduced to meet half of the cost of the tuberculosis service, the school medical service and the maternity and child welfare schemes, and a similar grant met three-quarters of the expenditure on venereal diseases schemes. Finally, in 1932, a grant, fixed in amount, was introduced to finance the provision by local authorities of free milk to necessitous children.

The Hospitals Trust Fund, an important new source of moneys for the health services, originated in the nineteenthirties.[2] The income of this Fund comes from sweepstakes on horse racing and it was used for capital expenditure and to pay deficits on the running expenses of voluntary hospitals. The Hospitals Commission was established to advise on issues from the Fund. During the period we are now discussing, expenditure from it was on a comparatively modest scale.

The Services in the Early Twentieth Century

The maternity and child welfare and school medical services
The services provided in the nineteenth century by the public authorities were designed to provide medical care for poor persons unable to provide such care for themselves and to protect the public from the spread of infectious diseases. The last decade of British rule was to see provision made by law for a new type of service. Under the Notification of Births (Extension) Act, 1915, sanitary authorities were given the simple power to 'make arrangements for attending to the health of ex-

---

[2]Under the Public Hospitals Act, 1933. See Chapter Seven.

pectant and nursing mothers and children under five years of age', and by the Public Health (Medical Treatment of Children) (Ireland) Act, 1919, county councils and county borough corporations were required to provide for the medical inspection and treatment of children attending national schools. The maternity and child welfare and school medical services which developed under these Acts widened the scope of the public health services far beyond their original definition in 1878. The introduction of these new services in Ireland represented the extension of a policy initiated for Britain.

The tuberculosis service

At the turn of the century, tuberculosis was becoming increasingly recognised as a disease which could be prevented and sometimes cured. The campaign by public authorities to eradicate it commenced in 1908, when county councils and county borough corporations were given power under the Tuberculosis Prevention (Ireland) Act to provide sanatoria and clinics and to operate tuberculosis schemes. This service was developed rather gradually and, although sanatoria were provided in most counties, there were never sufficient beds for tuberculosis cases before the Second World War.

The Services in the Period from 1922 to 1945

The new Department of Local Government and Public Health and the new local bodies which had evolved from the administrative tumult of the early twenties did not embark on the provision of any new health services. The old laws governing the scope and administration of these services continued to operate for over twenty years and any changes made during this period were of the nature of extensions and improvements in the facilities for making the services available.

The preventive services

The efficiency of the preventive services in the period following the change in administration was considerably improved by the appointment of the county medical officers of health. Hitherto the district medical officer of health had the basic responsibility for curbing outbreaks of infectious diseases in his dispensary district. His major preoccupation was rather with his work as dispensary doctor, and the serious outbreaks which were fairly frequent at the time usually called for much personal attention from the medical inspectors of the Department. The advantages of appointing a whole-time medical officer of health in each county to take charge of this work are obvious. The tuberculosis service and the school medical service and, in some areas, maternity and child welfare schemes, were developed in the twenties and thirties at a steady if unspectacular rate and this period also saw the introduction of diphtheria immunisation schemes.

Hospital services

The general hospitals were still administered under the Poor Relief Acts, but the spirit in which they were governed was changing. In the twenties other preoccupations had prevented any considerable activity in the building of hospitals, but the next decade saw the erection of some new county and district hospitals. Progressive improvements were made in the quality of the staffs of local authority hospitals, but increasing specialisation in medicine and surgery led to the development of the practice of public assistance authorities sending some patients to the voluntary hospitals in Dublin and elsewhere. On the other hand, patients not entitled to poor relief (or public assistance, as it became known under the Public Assistance Act, 1939, which consolidated the Poor Relief Acts), began increasingly to use the local authorities' hospitals as paying patients.

The dispensary medical service

Little change was made in the dispensary medical service during this period. This service was provided by the medical officers employed by the boards of health and public assistance in dispensaries and, where necessary, in the homes of the patients. Eligibility was determined by the issue of a red ticket, at the time the services of the doctor were needed, by a home assistance officer or warden appointed by the local authority. Maternity care was given under this service by the dispensary doctor and a midwife was employed for each dispensary district. Medicines were issued at the dispensary, generally by the dispensary doctor himself. By this time most of the dispensaries on which this service was centred were old buildings and they were lacking in comfort and often had inadequate facilities for treatment.

The 'additional benefits' scheme

This scheme was introduced in 1942 by the National Health Insurance Society, the body which then administered the national insurance scheme under which weekly cash benefits were paid to workers disabled through ill-health. Funds surplus to the Society's primary needs were made available to meet the whole or part of the cost to its members of hospital and specialist treatment (including appliances) and dental and optical treatment and appliances. The 'additional benefits' scheme operated separately from the local authority health services and it was limited to the expenditure of whatever remained after the claims for other benefits of the National Health Insurance Society had been met. It thus functioned intermittently and when the amount allocated to any of the additional benefits for any year was spent, the operation of that benefit ceased until the next year.

Chapter Three

The Period 1946 to 1960

The years immediately after the War, which brought a flood of plans and schemes for developments and changes in practically all sectors of public administration, nourished a considerable number of ideas for changes in and extensions of the health services. Dissatisfaction with the then existing services was due largely to three factors—the historical association of a large section of them with the Poor Law, the developments in medical science which made adequate hospital and specialist treatment too expensive for a middle class with incomes being steadily eroded by inflation and, of course, the developments taking place at the time in other countries, particularly Great Britain, where comprehensive services for the entire population were being planned. The most discussed of the plans put forward at the time was that of the late Most Reverend Dr. Dignan, Bishop of Clonfert. Under this plan, which was published in 1944, an improved and extended National Health Insurance Society would have been given the task of taking over and developing the services on an insurance basis. The Irish Medical Association, about the same time, published a scheme of health insurance to cater for the middle classes without extending the scope of State services. While neither of these schemes was accepted by the Government as meeting the needs of the time, their publication was indicative of the broad measure of agreement that something better was called for than what was then available. Elements of the ideas put forward in these schemes appeared in the later development of the services.

Administration

The Department of Health and other developments
The combination of local government and health in one department had brought a large number of wide-ranging services under one Minister. Many of these, not only on the health side,

19

stood in need of review after the War and, to permit of adequate attention being given to the impending changes in the health services, a separate Department of Health was established.[1] It became a separate entity in January 1947.

The functions of the Department of Health were defined in a White Paper[2] issued a little later as including 'the administration and business relating to the preparation, effective carrying out and co-ordination of measures conducive to the health of the people, including in particular measures for:

the prevention and cure of disease;

the treatment and care of persons suffering from physical defects or mental illnesses;

the regulation and control of the training and registration of persons for health services;

control over the appointment and conditions of service of appropriate local officers;

the initiation and direction of research;

ensuring that impure or contaminated food is not marketed and that adequate nutritive standards obtain in essential foodstuffs;

the control of proprietary medical and toilet preparations;

the registration of births, deaths and marriages; and

the collection, preparation, publication and dissemination of information and statistics relating to health.'

Responsibility for the water supplies, sewage disposal and other sanitary services remained with the Department of Local Government, it being agreed that the Department of Health would provide advice on the medical questions arising in the provision of these services. The distribution of functions between these Departments (and the Department of Social Welfare, which was also formed at this time) was effected by a series of Government orders which are listed in Appendix K.

---

[1] The new Department was established by the Ministers and Secretaries (Amendment) Act, 1946.
[2] *Outline of Proposals for the Improvement of the Health Services*, (Stationery C Office, Dublin, 1947).

A distinctive feature in the development of central administration in the period after 1945 was the extent to which consultative bodies, representative of vocational and other interests, were established to advise the Minister for Health. The most important of these was the National Health Council. This Council—whose present functions are described on page 49—was first established under the Health Act of 1947. The Minister, in constituting this Council, included nominees of a number of professional organisations but there was no obligation on him to do so. The Council met only when called together by the Minister and had authority to advise him only on subjects nominated by him. The Council's status was improved under the Health Act of 1953, when it was given authority, within limits, to meet of its own volition and to advise the Minister on subjects of its own choice; the 1953 Act also provided that at least half of the members be nominated by bodies representing the medical and ancillary professions and persons concerned with the management of voluntary hospitals. A number of specialist consultative councils were also appointed in this period.

Local administration

We have seen how the development of the local administration of the services had resulted in a number of different types of local authorities being concerned with the administration of health services. The trend in this period was towards a reduction in the numbers and types of authorities and towards the abolition of legal distinctions between different branches of the services. The first steps in this direction were taken under the Health Act of 1947. The simplification achieved under that Act was mainly in the transfer of responsibility for the preventive services in the urban districts (apart from the county boroughs) to the county councils. This meant that for diphtheria immunisation, infectious disease control, food hygiene and some other minor services, the number of responsible authorities was reduced from about ninety to thirty-one. As the county councils were also the public assistance authorities in most areas, the change made by this Act meant that in most areas one body was administering most of the health services.

The legal distinction between the services under the Health

Act and those administered by public assistance authorities remained until responsibility for the latter services was transferred to the 'health authorities' under the Health Act of 1953. Under that Act, the county and district hospitals which, as 'district institutions', were providing care under the public assistance authorities for 'poor persons unable by their own industry or other lawful means' to provide such care for themselves, joined the sanatoria in the category of 'health institutions' under the health authorities. The county council being both health authority and public assistance authority in most areas, this may not appear an important change, but it opened the way for more flexibility in the use of institutions.

This change in the legal status of the hospitals cleared the path for a definite break with the old Poor Law tradition in the government of these institutions. (It may surprise many to know that, up to 1954, the regulations[3] governing county homes and county and district hospitals were redolent of the Poor Law. These regulations stated, for example, that a person admitted as an 'inmate' 'shall, if circumstances so require and permit, before being placed in the appropriate part of the institution, be thoroughly cleansed, unless the medical officer of the institution otherwise directs, and be suitably clothed', that a person on admission might 'be searched for intoxicating liquor or other article, the introduction of which is prohibited by the public assistance authority' and that, as a concession, an 'inmate' might, 'if the matron or head nurse so approved, be permitted . . . to wear or use any clothing or other articles belonging to him'.) Whatever dubious reasons there might have been for such provisions in earlier times, clearly they had to go when the services in these hospitals were being made available to wider groups under the Act of 1953.

New local consultative health committees, including medical representatives, were set up under the Health Act of 1953. Their function was to advise the city and county managers on the operation of the general health services.

The net effect of the changes in the law on local administration under the Health Acts of 1947 and 1953 was that the county council, as health authority, administered all the health services, except for the mental treatment service, in most parts

---

[3]Public Assistance (General Regulations) Order 1942 (S. R. & O. No. 83 of 1942).

of the country. The administration of mental hospitals was still governed by a separate code (the Mental Treatment Act of 1945) and was in most areas in the hands of special joint boards.

In the Dublin, Cork, Limerick and Waterford areas, there remained complexes of health authorities, public assistance boards and mental hospital boards until, under the Health Authorities Act, 1960, there was established in each of these areas a unified authority with comprehensive responsibility for all the health services. These four unified health authorities were joint bodies within the local government system, the entire membership in each case being made up of local councillors nominated by the county and city council involved (and, in the case of the Dublin Health Authority, the Dun Laoghaire Borough Council).

By 1960, the number of the local authorities responsible for the health services had thus been reduced to twenty-seven (these four unified authorities and the county councils elsewhere). This was the culmination of the long trend towards having bigger and fewer local authorities responsible for health care: no further development within the local government system was to take place.

Finance

We have seen that in earlier periods the local rates, supplemented by modest State grants, were called upon to bear the cost of the health services. In 1947, the grants totalled about £830,000 and met 16 per cent of the total cost of the services. When, after the War, plans were prepared for substantial developments in the extensions of the services, it was clear that more generous financial assistance from the State would be needed. The White Paper issued in 1947 on the proposed extension of the services indicated that State subvention towards the cost would be substantially increased over the following years. Effect was given to this promise by the Health Services (Financial Provisions) Act, 1947. The basic principle of this Act was simple. The state undertook to meet, for each health authority, the full amount of any increase in the cost of its services until the total cost was twice the amount met by that authority from local taxation in the year to 31 March 1948. When the cost of the services rose above that level, it was to be divided equally between the rates and the Exchequer. In other words, the State paid for all increases until it was paying as much as the local authority and thereafter it met half of any increase. The object was to remove any financial grounds for lack of local enthusiasm for the development of the services.

The Services in the Period from 1945 to 1960

The tuberculosis service
The major endeavour in the years immediately after 1945 was in the development of the anti-tuberculosis services. An Act passed in 1945[4] permitted the Minister for Local Government and Public Health to arrange for the building of sanatoria. This was the first time since the workhouses were built by the Poor Law Commissioners that the central authority stepped outside its normal function of directing and co-ordinating the local services. Three sanatoria were provided under the Act—at Dublin, Cork and Galway—and were handed over, when completed, to the local authorities. In addition to the sanatoria erected under this Act, there was, during this period, widespread building and conversion of buildings from other uses by local health authorities. The number of beds available for tuberculosis became for the first time adequate for the demand.

The Health Act of 1947 made it clear that treatment in sanatoria was free for all and introduced the payment of maintenance allowances for dependants of persons undergoing treatment. All forms of tuberculosis became notifiable under this Act to the county or city medical officer (the old county medical officer of health or his city counterpart, under a different title): this helped considerably in the improvement of the service. These developments, coupled with the introduction of mass-radiography, BCG vaccination and new drugs, led to a gratifying drop in the number of deaths from tuberculosis and in the number of new cases being discovered.

Other preventive services
The law on the control of infectious diseases and on food

[4]The Tuberculosis (Establishment of Sanatoria) Act, 1945.

hygiene, which dated back to the Public Health (Ireland) Act, 1878, was codified and modernised under the Health Act of 1947. The main innovations in this code, which is contained in that Act and the Regulations made under it, were that free hospital treatment for infectious diseases became clearly available to all. The regulations to prevent the spread of infectious diseases from foreign-going ships were brought up to date and similar new regulations were introduced in relation to air traffic. The codification also involved the replacement of the provisions in the 1878 Act for the prevention of the sale of diseased or unsound food by the Food Hygiene Regulations of 1950.

Mental treatment
Up to 1945, nineteenth-century definitions, law and procedures still governed the services for the care of the mentally ill. Patients were 'committed' to mental hospitals on warrants signed by peace commissioners and there was provision for nothing between detention on such warrants and complete freedom, except for a system of 'trial discharge' which did not operate well in practice. Under the Mental Treatment Act of 1945, a more flexible procedure was introduced. It provided for patients being admitted on 'reception orders' signed by medical practitioners and for procedures for temporary and voluntary admissions to mental hospitals. The use of these considerably improved the working of the service.

Eligibility for mental hospital treatment continued to be based on the assistance principle until the Health Act of 1953 defined the classes eligible for this service as being the same as those entitled to general institutional and specialist services.

General hospital services
The services provided (mainly in county and district hospitals) by public assistance authorities became the General Institutional and Specialist Services under the Health Act of 1953. Eligibility was extended to a much wider class and became related not to individually-tested lack of means but to membership of one or other of four broadly-defined classes—persons insured for social welfare, persons with family incomes less than £600 a year, farmers with farms valued at or

under £50 and those outside these groups who could demonstrate 'undue hardship'. Some of these were entitled to the services without charge; statutory charges (originally six, later ten, shillings a day) were fixed for others and higher charges could be made for some of those brought in as hardship cases. Eligibility for out-patient specialist services was governed in a similar way. With the development of these services, the similar facilities under the 'additional benefits' scheme of the Department of Social Welfare described on page 18 were withdrawn. The development of the new service, particularly in the Dublin area, involved an increased acceptance by local authorities of responsibility for the cost of treatment of patients in voluntary hospitals. The income limit of £600 was raised to £800 in 1958, to make allowance for the fall in the value of money since 1953.

Maternity and child care
The maternity and child care services prior to 1953 comprised attendance by dispensary medical officers and midwives on poor patients (with hospital care for them if necessary), and clinics and nursing services provided by health authorities or voluntary agencies in some areas. These services were considerably extended under the Health Act of 1953. Women in (or dependent on persons in) the four groups eligible for hospital services became entitled to a full maternity service, with choice of doctor and midwife and, under some financial penalty, choice of hospital or maternity home. Comprehensive medical and nursing care for their infants was also provided for. Maternity cash grants of £4 for each birth were introduced for women in what became known as the lower income group. A requirement on health authorities to provide child welfare clinic services was substituted for the permission to do so which was given to them under earlier law and new regulations were made for the improvement of the school health services.

Other services
A number of the other services were affected by the changes made under the Health Act of 1953. The dispensary service and the dispensary doctors were transferred from the public assistance code to the health authorities; a better system of

recording entitlement to this service replaced the issue of 'red tickets'; dental, ophthalmic and aural services for the lower income group and for children were continued and the extension of these services to other groups was envisaged; a more liberal code for the governing of county homes was introduced; provision was made for the development of a comprehensive rehabilitation service; health authorities were required to pay allowances to disabled persons and the law on the boarding-out of children by local authorities was improved.

General policy on services
The policy which evolved from this period and to which concrete expression was given in the Health Act of 1953 can be summarised as providing for each class the services which the persons in it could not themselves afford. Thus, the general practitioner service remained available only to those who could individually demonstrate need, and the institutional services, being more costly, were provided for a wider group. Apart from the extension of the latter services to a greater proportion of the population, the main change in them lay in the statutory specification of the general groups eligible, in place of the previous individual assessment of need. A broad-spectrum means test replaced the unpalatable assistance basis of the earlier services. Once a person could show that he was in one of the statutory groups, his entitlement became independent of an official's judgement on his need for the service.

Before leaving the 1953 Act, it is as well to quote the following extract, which sets out the principle underlying the provision of services under it.

'4 (1) Nothing in this Act or any instrument thereunder shall be construed as imposing an obligation on any person to avail himself of any service provided under this Act or to submit himself or any person for whom he is responsible to health examination or treatment.

(2) Any person who avails himself of any service provided under this Act shall not be under any obligation to submit himself or any person for whom he is responsible to a health examination or treatment which is contrary to the teaching of his religion'.

This section still remains in force.

Voluntary health insurance

The statutory health services offered little to those in the upper income group. An advisory body was set up in 1956 to examine the feasibility of a State-sponsored voluntary health insurance scheme to meet the needs of this group. Arising out of the Report of this body[5] a Bill was introduced which became the Voluntary Health Insurance Act, 1957. This Act set up a board to operate voluntary health insurance schemes, mainly for hospital care, on a non-profit making basis. The public response was good. By the end of 1958, the Board's various schemes covered a total of some 57,000 people.

[5]See Chapter Nine.

Chapter Four

The Period Since 1961

Since 1961 much has been said and written on the health services. A select committee of Dáil Éireann on the services sat from 1962 to 1965, a Government White Paper outlining future policy was published in January 1966, and several advisory bodies submitted reports during these three years. These reports are listed in the bibliography and this list shows the range of subjects specially examined in this period.

It was a period of scrutiny of existing services, of identification of problems, and of recommendations—sometimes contradictory—for solutions. It was a period of uncertainty for some existing services pending decisions on changes. It was a period of new medical discoveries and of a change in emphasis in the aims of the health services, because of the decline in some former problems, the magnification of others and the emergence of some new ones. Heart disease, cancer, psychiatric conditions (including those associated with alcoholism and drug dependence), diseases associated with ageing and accidents emerged as the main concerns for the nineteen-seventies. Just as was the case with tuberculosis in earlier times, these were problems rooted in the way of life of the people, but because the way of life had become so much more complex, solutions to these problems were clearly going to be much more difficult to find.

The years since 1961 have seen a realisation and acceptance of the fact that the increasing fruits of medical science could not easily be made available to all who could benefit from them and that, because of the complexity of modern medical organisation, changes and new involvements in health administration were called for. This was a period too within which the awesome nature of the financial problem of the health services became evident, not only in this country. The need for ordered priorities in the health expenditure became more apparent.

The period saw the passage of the Health Act, 1970 and the Health Contributions Act, 1971. These Acts offered solutions to some of the problems outlined without, however, any pretence that perfect solutions were possible in an imperfect world.

Administration

Central administration

Perhaps the most noteworthy event in central administration was the publication in 1969 of the report of the Public Services Organisation Review Group (the Devlin Report), which dealt with the reorganisation of Government Departments generally. The essential recommendation of this report was that Ministers should divest themselves of direct executive responsibility for services, so as to be free to concentrate on the general planning, organisation and review of services. The report recognised that organisational developments in the health services had been in accordance with this recommendation and a restructuring of the Department of Health on the principles of the report was accomplished during the period.

An important Act was passed in 1961[1] to allow the Minister to set up corporate bodies to operate particular health services not suitable for localised operation. Several bodies were set up under this Act during the period. Among them were the Medico-Social Research Board, the National Drugs Advisory Board and the Health Education Bureau. Another Act[2] transferred former workhouse lands to the local authorities and, in 1971, the administration of the Central Mental Hospital at Dundrum was transferred from the Department of Health to the newly established Eastern Health Board.[3] Both of these moves were in accord with the general policy to devolve detailed executive work from the Department.

The Minister's powers to set up advisory bodies were widely used during this period. In addition, the National Health Council continued to exercise its function of examining and

[1] The Health (Corporate Bodies) Act, 1961. A full list of the bodies set up under the Act is given in Appendix A.

[2] The State Lands (Workhouses) Act, 1962.

[3] Under section 44 of the Health Act, 1970 and the Central Mental Hospital Order, 1971.

reporting on the services (and, indeed, on the reports of the several other advisory bodies). In 1972, there was an important change for the hospital services in the establishment of Comhairle na nOspidéal, an independent body to govern the creation of new consultant medical posts in hospitals and to advise generally on hospital services.

Local administration

The local authority administration described earlier remained in control of the services until March 1971: new health boards set up under the Health Act, 1970, took over on that date. The idea of taking health administration away from the local authorities was not new. The White Paper published in 1947 tentatively put forward a proposal for special bodies directly responsible to the Minister for Health to administer the health services, with provision for regional co-ordination, but this proposal was not followed up at the time. The idea of special bodies for the administration of the health services surfaced again in the 1966 White Paper, in which it was proposed that legislation should be introduced to transfer health administration from the existing local authorities to regional boards whose membership would 'represent a partnership between local government, central government and the vocational organisations'.

One might ask why there was such a long gestation period for what might seem to be an obvious move, viz. to split locally what had been split centrally when Health and Local Government were made into separate Departments of State in 1947. The answer may be that there was a reluctance to take health administration away from the local government system because, whatever doubt there might have been about the effectiveness of the local authorities in the nineteen-forties, it was clear, once the county management system had settled down, that the county councils and other health authorities provided, within the confines of the counties, a good system of administration and one which should not be tampered with without very good reason. It is clear from the 1966 White Paper that the eventual decision to take health administration away from the local authorities was not lightly reached. The White Paper stated:

'126. Notwithstanding the strong case for changing the administration of the health services in this way the Government would not wish the change to be made if there were a danger that the transfer from them of their health functions would so diminish the scope of the local authorities' work that they would become ineffectual bodies evoking little interest in the community. This danger is not real. If the existing local authorities lose the direct administration of the health services, which now makes up about one-third of their total activities, they will still remain, beneath the Government itself, probably the most important administrative organs in the State. Shorn of their health functions, the county councils would but be restored, as respects the scope of their work, to what they were in the nineteen-thirties, as health services of our present-day scope are quite a recent addition to their functions. The local councils will retain responsibility for the general planning and development of their areas, for the improvement and maintenance of the roads system, for housing development, for sanitary services and for several other general local government functions. The local government services are all developing and it is, indeed, better that local councils and county managers should in future be able to give them their undivided attention.'

The case for the change in health administration, as stated in the White Paper, had two bases. The first was that, because the State had taken over the major financial interest in the health services and this interest was increasing, it was desirable that a new administrative framework combining national and local interests should be developed for the services. The second basis for a change arose from the developments in professional techniques and equipment, which meant that better services could be provided on an inter-county basis. This argument was, of course, of greater relevance in the hospital services. For many of these services, and for the general organisation of hospital services, the county had become too small as a unit. In 1966, over half of all in-patients in acute hospitals were being treated in the regional and teaching hospitals in the larger centres, and specialist services at out-patient departments were being organised increasingly on a regional basis. It had become clear that the future efficiency of the hospital services was becoming more and more dependent on full co-ordination of the various units and that a board covering a number of counties could plan and arrange the hospital services for those counties so as to better serve the people in its area.

From many counties, hundreds of patients were being sent annually at the expense of the local health authority to hospitals in other areas, but in these circumstances, the county concerned had no say in the organisation or operation of these hospitals. The grouping of counties under new bodies, representative of all counties within the group, meant that each county could become directly associated with the hospital centres to which most of its patients were traditionally sent and have a voice in the creation of policy on the services in those centres.

On these arguments, the case was made for the organisation of the hospital services in larger units. The option was open to do this and to leave the operation of the other health services, such as the general practitioner service and the preventive service, with the local authorities. This option was, however, rejected because always in mind as the main consideration was the importance of unitary control and responsibility for all the health services in each area. The services are all interdependent. Hospital care is related to what general practitioners do and may often be an alternative to general practitioner care, and, of course, the activities of the preventive services can also affect the requirements for hospital and other services. It was, therefore, decided that it would be an essential principle of the new administration that one body would be responsible in each of the areas chosen for the operation of all the health services.

It was, in any event, apparent that many of the health services outside hospitals—such as general practitioner services, the public health nursing services and child welfare services—would benefit from being organised across county boundaries. A surprising number of our cities and towns straddle county boundaries (examples are Limerick, Waterford, Ballinasloe, Clonmel, Drogheda, Carrick-on-Suir and New Ross). With inter-county administration, such towns can more effectively be used as bases for these services. It was apparent too that larger units of administration would allow for the more economic employment of social workers and other staff for the child care and geriatric services.

Following the publication of the 1966 White Paper, the proposals were widely discussed with the local authorities and other bodies and following these discussions, a decision was taken to proceed with the legislation to set up the new health boards. While no decision was then taken on the number of boards, it was thought that about six to eight health boards would be appropriate.

The impact of the Fitzgerald Report

The publication in June 1968 of the report of the Consultative Council on the General Hospital Services (the Fitzgerald Report) influenced further thought on these proposals. This report was concerned mainly with the sizes and kinds of hospitals needed to meet modern requirements, but the consultative council also made recommendations on administration, which would have left the control of hospital services separate from that of the other health services. It recommended an administrative system for the hospitals with a central body to control the distribution of specialties and the allocation of consultants, with three regional hospital boards based on the medical teaching centres of Dublin, Cork and Galway (in which hospitals would be vested) and with special management committees for individual hospitals or groups of hospitals. For the reasons outlined above this separate system of administration did not commend itself, but it was accepted that special co-ordinating bodies would be desirable for the hospital services. It was accordingly decided to set up three regional hospital boards based on the medical teaching centres and with functions 'in relation to the general organisation and development of hospital services in an efficient and satisfactory manner in the hospitals administered by health boards and other bodies in its functional area which are engaged in the provision of services under the Health Acts'.

The Health Act, 1970

The Health Bill, 1969, included provisions for setting up the health boards and the regional hospital boards and for the dissolution of bodies which would become redundant because of the changes, including the Dublin, Cork, Limerick and Waterford Health Authorities and the Hospitals Commission.

The Bill was introduced in January 1969: it had the distinction of being moved at the special commemorative session of the Fiftieth Anniversary of the First Dáil in the Mansion House, Dublin. It received a second reading in the following May but its course was interrupted by the 1969 general election. After the election, the Bill was re-activated at Committee stage by special resolution of the Dáil. It became law in February 1970.

The provisions in the Health Act, 1970 for establishing the new administrative system were broadly framed, leaving the details on the number and constitution of the health boards for subsequent regulations. This type of provision was preferred, so that the debate on the Bill would relate to the principle of whether or not the health boards and other bodies should be established, without becoming involved in the details of the system. However, so that the Houses of the Oireachtas would later have an opportunity of approving or rejecting the detailed proposals, it was provided in the Act that the regulations setting up the health boards would be subject to approval by resolutions of each House.

Proposals for the grouping of counties and for the constitutions of the health boards were circulated to the local authorities concerned in September 1969, and the Minister held preliminary discussions with representatives of the authorities in the autumn of that year. The Minister's proposals were then put into final form and submitted to the Dáil and Seanad in May 1970. The draft regulations were subsequently approved by both Houses and were made in July. The Regulations came into effect on 1 October 1970, so that the boards were legally established then. The process of appointing members was completed in November and the first meetings of the boards were held shortly after. However, the boards did not become responsible for the operation of the health services until 1 April, 1971.

Meanwhile, steps were in train for the recruitment of the chief executive officers for the new boards. The Act allowed the Minister to initiate this before the boards were actually established and recruitment proceeded, through the Local Appointments Commissioners, during the summer of 1970. Most of the chief executive officers had been selected and were available to the boards before they met. The majority of them came from the local authority service.

The 1970 Act also provided for the establishment of local committees, for the purpose of maintaining contact at county level with the operation of the health services. These committees are mainly advisory and their meetings are attended by the chief executive officer or another senior officer of the health board.

Finance

Up to 1966, the financial arrangements described in Chapter 3 continued to apply. The Health Services Grant from the Exchequer met 50 per cent of the cost of the services provided by the local authorities and the balance was met from local sources (the 'local sources', in fact, included some further state aid towards reducing the rates on agriculture and land; this complication is referred to again in Chapter 7). A review of the existing financial system was included in the 1966 White Paper. Having referred to the continuing trends towards increasing costs and having given estimates for the improvements and modifications in the services as then being proposed, the White Paper went on to state:

'116. *The Government, having studied this issue, are satisfied that the local rates are not a form of taxation suitable for collecting additional money on this scale. They propose, therefore, that the cost of the further extensions of the services should not be met in any proportion by the local rates.* Following this decision, other possible sources of revenue to meet the additional costs are being considered but it seems likely that the general body of central taxation must bear the major part of the burden. *Pending further consideration of the methods by which extensions of the health services will be financed in future years, the Government have decided to make arrangements which will ensure that the total cost of the services falling on local rates in respect of the year 1966-67 will not exceed the cost in respect of the year 1965-66.'*

The 'freeze' on the rates contribution was not continued in

full for succeeding years but grants supplementary to the statutory 50 per cent were paid so as to reduce the impact on the rates of the continuing rise in health expenditure. By 1970, the State grants specifically towards the health services were meeting 56 per cent of the total cost. The financial arrangements for the new health boards put these arrangements for supplementary grants on a formal basis. In 1973, the Government decided that the contribution from the rates to the cost of the health services would be phased out entirely. This move was completed by 1977, so that there is now no contribution from the rates towards the cost of the services. This is the culmination of the trend initiated thirty years before.

Paragraph 116 of the White Paper had referred to 'other possible sources of revenue' being considered. Among these sources was a scheme of contributions by eligible persons. Such a scheme was introduced in October, 1971: it is described in Chapter 7.

The Services in the Period since 1961

No fundamental change was made in the structure of the services before 1971. Rather was this a time of development of the policy of the previous period, as described in the last chapter. Indeed, the Government, in the 1966 White Paper, emphasised that it favoured further development on the existing lines. The White Paper stated:

'16. By following this broad principle, there has been a more effective use of the necessarily limited proportion of the national product which can be devoted to the public development of health services than if an effort had been made to develop on a much broader base a scheme with the features of a comprehensive free-for-all national health service. The present services meet the essential needs of the population: insofar as it is now proposed to make changes in them, these changes are justified in each case by special consideration.'

The general medical service
The origin and nature of the dispensary system has been referred to in previous chapters. The White Paper assessed this

service and proposed a radical reorganisation in the following terms:

'41. The dispensary system has many merits. It ensures that everywhere, even in the most remote western districts, there will normally be at least one highly qualified and experienced medical practitioner to provide services for the lower income group (and, incidentally, for the rest of the people through his private practice). It provides all needed drugs, medicines and appliances for those in that group at no cost to them and at a moderate cost to public funds. That there is now considerable advocacy for replacing this service by one of a different kind does not detract from the quality of the service itself, nor reflect in any way on the work of the dispensary doctors who, for over a century, have been the strong foundation of our health services for the lower income group. But, with all its advantages, the dispensary system has one feature which must lead to its re-appraisal in any broad review of the health services in the context of social development: that is, that one who uses the service is set apart from a person who arranges for private medical care, in that he attends at the dispensary and not the doctor's private surgery, and has no choice of doctor. In assessing broadly the merits of the dispensary system, this feature must be accepted as outweighing the system's advantages and, now that many projects of greater priority in the improvement of our services have been completed or are well advanced, the time has come when it is possible to consider replacing this system by one more akin to what is arranged privately by those outside the lower income group.

42. *The Government propose, therefore, that the general practitioner service organised by the health authorities should be re-arranged so that those whose medical care is paid for by the health authorities will be able to get the same kind of service as others can now get through private arrangement. This proposal involves substituting for the dispensary service a service with the greatest practicable choice of doctor and the least practicable distinction between private patients and those availing themselves of the service.'*

The White Paper also stated that, in the context of a scheme for a choice of doctor, it would be preferable if drugs were supplied through the retail chemists (or the doctors themselves where this was not practicable).

The implementation of these proposals had to await the enactment of the Health Act, 1970, and negotiations with the medical and pharmaceutical organisations on the details of the arrangements were protracted. The new general medical service based on these proposals commenced in the Eastern Health Board area on 1 April 1972 and in the rest of the country on 1 October 1972. It is described in Chapter 10.

Services in hospitals and homes
Hospitals were becoming increasingly complex organisations, offering a wider range of skills for the diagnosis and treatment of diseases. As these skills became more sophisticated and specialised, increasing emphasis was called for on effective planning of hospital services, and the avoidance of duplication and unnecessarily prolonged stay in hospitals. The Fitzgerald Report emphasised these points and recommended solutions to the problems involving a concentration of specialised hospital services in fewer centres.

New drugs and new methods of treatment for the mentally ill changed the pattern of care dramatically. There was an increased emphasis on out-patient treatment and the proportion of patients in mental hospitals who entered voluntarily had increased substantially. There was a large increase in the accommodation for the mentally handicapped and the facilities for them were improved in many respects.

Care of the aged
There was an increased recognition of the special problems of the aged and of the need to develop specialised services for them. A number of other Government Departments and agencies are involved in this and the responsibility for co-ordinating activities was assigned to the Minister for Health and his Department. In 1971, the National Social Service Council was set up by the Minister to co-ordinate the activities of voluntary agencies and public authorities. The 1970 Health Act provided for the establishment of home help services. Registration of

homes in which old people are maintained for profit was provided for in 1964.[4]

Preventive services

Perhaps the most noteworthy development was in the fluoridation of water supplies. This measure to prevent dental caries was provided for in the Health (Fluoridation of Water Supplies) Act, 1960. After an interesting, long-drawn-out but unsuccessful effort to have this Act declared unconstitutional by the courts, it was progressively implemented throughout the country and piped public water supplies are now mainly fluoridated. Another notable new preventive measure was the highly successful oral poliomyelitis vaccination campaign in 1965. Following on this campaign, poliomyelitis has been almost eliminated from the community.

The period also saw a widening realisation of the need for further measures to protect the public from danger in the sale and distribution of drugs and poisons. The Poisons Act, 1961, gave the Minister wider powers to make regulations on this and the Misuse of Drugs Act, 1977, gave better powers to control the abuse of drugs of addiction. Plans for improvements in the child health services were pushed ahead, the aim being to replace the child welfare clinic schemes and the school health examination service with a comprehensive well-planned service offering surveillance from infancy to the conclusion of primary schooling.

In the last few years there has been heightened emphasis on positive measures in the field of prevention. Health education has been given a more prominent role, particularly in relation to smoking and alcohol-related diseases. The Tobacco Products (Control of Advertising, Sponsorship and Sales Promotion) Act, 1979, gives the Minister for Health wide powers to restrict advertising of tobacco products.

Other services

The Health Act, 1970, provided for improvements and adjustments in a number of other services. In-patient and out-patient hospital care for a number of long-term conditions in children was made available free to all and drugs for certain long-term

[4]Under the Health (Homes for Incapacitated Persons) Act, 1964.

ailments were also made available without means test.

Eligibility
The 1970 Act codified the earlier provisions on eligibility for the services, making some beneficial adjustments. The income limit for hospital services, which had been increased to £1,200 a year in 1966 to £1,600 in 1971, was raised to £2,250 a year in April 1974 and to £3,000 a year in 1976.

Voluntary health insurance
The Voluntary Health Insurance Board flourished during this period. The number of persons covered by the Board's scheme increased from 78,778 in February, 1960 to 645,165 in February, 1978, the scheme of benefits was made more flexible and otherwise improved and the Board became the accepted agency whereby those not covered by the public services could insure themselves against the increasing costs of ill-health. Indeed, many of those entitled to use the public authorities' services invested in supplementary cover from the Voluntary Health Insurance Board to enable them to have private or semi-private treatment.

Developments in April 1979
A considerable widening of the coverage of some services — mainly the hospital services — came into effect in April 1979. This was tied in with the commencement of a scheme of pay-related health contributions. Broadly, hospital-based services in public wards became available to all free of charge, except for consultants' fees in the case of those over the 'cut-off' point for health contributions, which was fixed at £5,500 a year. At the same time, the Voluntary Health Insurance Board re-cast its schemes so as to complement effectively the new arrangements for eligibility. These developments are referred to in more detail in later chapters.

*   *   *

This and the preceding chapters have been concerned with the origins of and the mutations and developments in the efforts of public authorities to care for the health of the people. The limitations of the work, which specified that the account should be descriptive with little commentary, might lead a reader to assume that the changes described just happened, smoothly and with no great effort of will. They did not, of course. The services, in recent decades at any rate, were forged by much public debate and some political controversy. It is for others to deal with the history of this, but it is fitting for the author to conclude these chapters by listing the Ministers for Health who have been responsible for the establishment of the modern services and whom he, as one of those in the Department of Health, has had the privilege to serve. The office seemed to attract distinguished holders: once it was held by the Taoiseach and on three occasions by the Tánaiste.

The list is
January 1947 to February 1948—Dr James Ryan, TD
February 1948 to April 1951—Dr Noel Browne, TD
April 1951 to June 1951—Mr John A. Costello, TD
June 1951 to June 1954—Dr James Ryan, TD
June 1954 to March 1957—Mr Thomas F. O'Higgins, TD
March 1957 to April 1965—Mr Sean MacEntee, TD
April 1965 to July 1966—Mr Donogh O'Malley, TD
July 1966 to July 1969—Mr Sean Flanagan, TD
July 1969 to March 1973—Mr Erskine Childers, TD
March 1973 to July 1977—Mr Brendan Corish, TD
July 1977 to date—Mr Charles J. Haughey, TD.

Chapter Five

Organisation

The power to decide what health services there will be and how they will be administered does not reside in any one person or institution. Basically, of course, the civil authority for the provision of the services comes from the legislature. It flows mainly through the Minister for Health but, in substantial volume, it passes on to the several functional bodies concerned in the provision of the services. They in their turn, together with special advisory bodies, may influence the source of this flow—generally in an indirect fashion through the Minister. The diagram below illustrates the administration.

Fig. 1 **ADMINISTRATION OF THE HEALTH SERVICE**

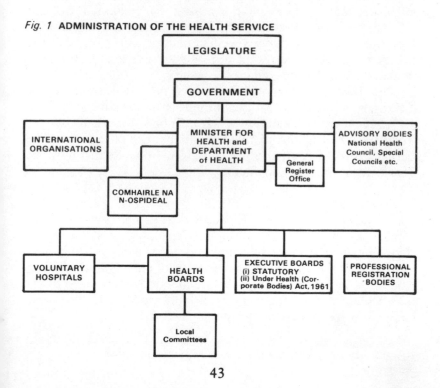

Central Administration

The Legislature[1]

The legal basis for the health services is contained in the Acts passed by the Dáil and Seanad, and the actions of all the other organs of administration must conform with those Acts. In general, the Acts governing the provision of the health services (and notably the Health Acts of 1947, 1953 and 1970) do not lay down in detail how the services will operate but leave this to regulations made by the Minister, to guidelines and directives issued by his Department and to the decisions of the health boards and other executive agencies.

The Minister, in preparing regulations, cannot do anything which the parent Act does not provide for, nor can he assume powers by regulations which he has not otherwise been given. The content of regulations is subject to control by the legislature. In a few instances, a draft must be approved by the Dáil and Seanad before the regulations are made. Where this does not apply the regulations must be presented to both Houses after they are made and either House may, by resolution, annul them within a specified period. This control is one which is unlikely to be used but its existence is a curb on the making of regulations of doubtful validity.

The Dáil also exercises a control on the actions of the Minister by its debates on the annual Estimates for the Department of Health. In addition, each member of the Dáil has the right to ask questions of the Minister on the operation of the services and, if he wishes, to initiate a fuller discussion if he thinks the reply is unsatisfactory.

The Government

As in the case of the other branches of the public services, decisions on the initiation of health legislation rests with the Government. So do other major decisions on health policy. These are normally taken on the basis of submissions made by the Minister for Health and, before any decision is taken by the Government, any other minister concerned will have considered the proposal from his point of view.

[1]A detailed account of the working of the legislature is given in *The Houses of the Oireachtas* by J. C. Smyth (Institute of Public Administration,1964).

The Minister for Health and his Department

Most of the powers given to the Minister for Health relate to the making of statutory regulations and orders and to the general supervision of the activities of the health boards and other executive agencies in the provision of health services. As the co-ordinating and supervising authority for the services, the Minister's functions range from approving the general pattern to control of the method of appointment, the remuneration and the conditions of service of health personnel. The Minister does not have any power to give directions on the eligibility of individual persons for health services or on how the services are to be made available to individuals. Such decisions are left to the subordinate agencies.

By a tradition going back to the times of the Poor Law administration, the exercise of the Minister's controls has involved a considerable number of detailed approvals or 'sanctions' for specific actions of local bodies. The transfer of administration to the eight health boards led to a review of the methods by which the overall supervision of the services is effected. More emphasis is placed on control by way of general guidelines and directives, coupled with budgetary controls, in place of many of the individual approvals called for in the past. The Health Act, 1970, and the regulations made under it were designed to permit this.

Statutory powers are vested in the Minister. Decisions on the use of these powers are his responsibility, but, in accordance with the Ministers and Secretaries Acts, the Department of Health is there to deal with the 'departmental administration' relative to the Minister's functions. This 'departmental administration' is, in fact, the taking of whatever action is necessary (and which is, of course, permitted by law) to execute the decisions on policy made by the Minister. The Department also provides information and advice to the Minister on questions arising for his decision.

The head of the Department is the Secretary, who has overall administrative control of the Department and has the main responsibility for seeing that the Minister's policies are carried out. The Secretary is also charged personally with responsibility for ensuring that all payments made from the Department's Vote are legally and properly made for purposes covered by the Vote. He must, therefore, be especially careful to warn the Minister if he thinks that any expenditure which the latter directs is not covered by the Vote for Health.

The organisation of the Department of Health is arranged in accordance with the principles set out in the Report of the Public Services Organisation Review Group.[2] The report proposed that each Department should be re-arranged so as to separate policy-making from executive functions. The Department of Health was the first to be re-organised on this basis.

The policy-making component in a Department restructured in this way is called the Aireacht and, in accordance with the PSORG Report, it is made up of 'staff' units and 'line' divisions. The staff units are for planning, finance, organisation and personnel. In addition, because of the strong professional input required in the Department of Health, the Chief Medical Officer and other professional staff retain a separate status within the Aireacht. The 'line' divisions of the Aireacht are in two groups, one for community services and one for hospital services.

The role of the Department of Health has always been mainly in the field of policy making and the execution of policies in the health services is almost entirely left to the outside agencies described later in this Chapter. The only executive units within the Department are the office of the Registrar-General for Births, Deaths and Marriages, the Hospital Planning Office (which co-operates with executive agencies in the design and building of hospitals) and a section dealing with a superannuation scheme for voluntary hospitals.

The PSORG Report envisaged that in each Aireacht a management advisory committee should be constituted to advise the Secretary in formulating proposals for the Minister. The Management Advisory Committee in the Department of Health consists basically of the Secretary, the Chief Medical Officer and the Assistant Secretaries. Heads of other units and other members of the professional staff may also be asked to attend meetings of the committee.[3]

---

[2]Report of Public Services Organisation Review Group, 1966-1969 (Prl 792)

[3]This new structure followed, with some changes, the report of a 1973 Task Force 'Restructuring the Department of Health the Separation of Policy and Executive' (Prl 3445).

Co-ordination of Hospital Services

Because they were designed to share with the Minister and his Department the function of controlling and co-ordinating the hospital services, it is logical to deal next with the special bodies established under Section 41 of the Health Act, 1970. These are Comhairle na nOspidéal (the Hospital Council) and three regional hospital boards. These bodies were not designed to be concerned with the administration of the services, in that they were not charged with the day-to-day administration of hospitals; their function was specified to lie rather in co-ordinating and controlling the development of the services in both the hospitals managed by the health boards and those hospitals owned and managed by voluntary bodies which provide services under the Health Acts.

Comhairle na nOspidéal and the three regional hospital boards were established on 1 July, 1972 under the Health (Hospital Bodies) Regulations, 1972.

Comhairle na nOspidéal

The primary functions of Comhairle na nOspidéal are concerned with regulating the numbers and types of consultant appointments in hospitals taking patients under the Health Acts and with specifying qualifications for the appointment of consultants. It is also the general advisory body on hospital services and it is expected that it will become involved in arranging the selection of consultants.[4]

Under the Act, at least half of the members of the Comhairle must be 'registered medical practitioners engaged in a consultant capacity in the provision of hospital services'. The regulations provide for twenty-seven members, of whom at least fourteen are in this category. The other appointees include officers of the Department of Health and persons involved in voluntary hospitals and in the health boards. The chairman and vice-chairman of the Comhairle are selected by the Minister from amongst the members. The Comhairle has authority to establish committees and has used this authority widely.

[4]The exact specification of the Comhairle's functions is given in section 41(1) of the Act.

Regional hospital boards

The 1970 Act required that three regional hospital boards, based on Dublin, Cork and Galway would be established to perform 'such functions as may be prescribed in relation to the general organisation and development of hospital services in an efficient and satisfactory manner in the hospitals administered by health boards and other bodies in its functional area which are engaged in the provision of services under this Act'. The Minister's regulations spelt out the detailed functions of these bodies. The functions included examining estimates, governing numbers and kinds of personnel, allocating capital resources in the region and providing management advisory services. It was intended that the regional hospital boards would take over from the Department of Health and from the Hospitals Commission many of their functions on the control and co-ordination of hospital services.

Under the Act, one half of the members of a regional hospital board are appointed by the health boards whose functional areas are included in that of the regional hospital board. The other half of the members are appointed by the Minister 'after consultation with, or on the nomination of, such bodies representative of persons concerned with the provision of hospital services and such other bodies (including bodies engaged in medical education) as the Minister considers appropriate'.

In the event, the regional hospital boards did not have a significant role in hospital policy. For some time it has been recognised that, with the developing roles of the Comhairle and the health boards, the regional hospital boards are unnecessary. They remain in legal existence, however, for the time being.

Advisory Bodies

The Minister for Health and his Department have many sources of advice. On broad policy issues, there is, of course, a steady stream of opinion from parliamentary debates and, on more detailed points, the Minister, in the normal course of his political activity, will see a reflection of public opinion in what is said and written to him. There are also many contacts, of different degrees of formality, by the Minister and Departmental officers with representative members of the health professions and with those involved in the health board administration. Advice is available on a more institutionalised basis from a number of bodies.

The National Health Council

The function of the National Health Council is 'to advise the Minister on such general matters affecting or incidental to the health of the people as may be referred to them by the Minister and on such other general matters (other than conditions of employment of officers and servants and the amount of payment of grants and allowances) relating to the operation of the health services as they think fit'.[5] The Council is appointed by the Minister for Health but at least half of the members must be 'nominated by bodies representative of the medical and ancillary professions and of persons concerned with the management of voluntary hospitals'. The selection of the other members of the Council rests with the Minister but it has been the practice for him to include persons involved in other bodies concerned with health questions, such as the trade union organisations. The members of the Council go out of office every two years.

The National Health Council appoints its own chairman and regulates its own procedure but, if it wishes to meet more than three times in any quarter, it must seek the consent of the Minister. An officer of the Department of Health acts as secretary to the Council. Its meetings are held in private.

The Minister is required to seek the Council's advice before he makes regulations under the Health Acts or the Mental Treatment Acts. If, because of urgency, the Minister cannot arrange this before he makes the regulations, he is obliged to ask for the Council's advice on them after they have been made. Advising on regulations, however, forms only part of the Council's work. It has concerned itself with and reported on practically all the major developments in the health services which have been considered since it was reconstituted in its present form in 1954.

The Council presents an annual report to the Minister and he is obliged to publish it, with any comments which he wishes.

[5] Section 41 of the Health Act, 1953.

The reports of the Council for recent years show the result of its discussions on the many recent changes in health policy. The Council advised on the choice of doctor scheme, on the proposals for regional administration of the health services, on the organisation of ambulance services, on family planning and on a number of other topics.

Other advisory bodies

A host of special advisory bodies exists. They are of two kinds, standing statutory advisory bodies and special bodies set up from time to time to advise on specific problems. The former group includes Comhairle na nOspidéal, the Medico-Social Research Board, the National Drugs Advisory Board and the statutory professional registration bodies.

There have been very many special advisory bodies in the health field. The constitution of such bodies can range from a formal Commission of Enquiry (as in the case of the Mental Illness Commission, 1964), through a consultative council set up by statutory instrument, to informal working parties. Practically all aspects of the health services have at one time or another been covered by investigations by bodies of these kinds. The reports of various advisory bodies which influenced recent health policy are referred to on page 29: these and other reports are included in the bibliography. Included among the informal working parties was one with representatives of the medical profession which worked out the details of the 'choice of doctor' scheme.

Local Executive Bodies

Health boards

The organs of central administration mentioned above are mainly concerned with broad questions of health policy, of the scope of the services and of how they should be organised. The main burden of work in operating the services decreed by these central authorities is laid on the health boards.

Section 4(1) of the Health Act, 1970, provided—

'For the administration of the health services in the State, the Minister shall, after consultation with the Minister for Local Government, by regulations establish such number of boards (to be known and in this Act referred to as health boards) as may appear to him to be appropriate, and by such regulations shall specify the title and define the functional area of each health board so established and, subject to sub-section (2), shall specify the membership of each health board.'

Section 4(2) specified in broad terms the constitution of each health board. The majority of the members must be appointed by the local county councils and county borough councils (and, in the appropriate case, the Corporation of Dun Laoghaire) and the remainder of the membership must include persons elected by medical practitioners and members of ancillary professions. Under section 4(4), consultations with the county councils and other nominating local authorities were required before regulations were made under the section.

Each health board set up under the Act is a body corporate, with the usual authority to hold and dispose of land, etc. The Act contains rules relating to the membership and meetings of the boards and provisions allowing them to set up committees (to which functions may be delegated), to act jointly in providing services (including, if necessary, the establishment of a joint body) and to co-operate with local authorities. The boards can also enter into arrangements with other bodies, such as voluntary hospitals, to provide services on their behalf.

Eight such boards were set up under the Health Boards Regulations, 1970. The table on page 52 sets out the areas served by these boards and the constitution of each of them.

In designing this structure, a number of factors were taken into account. Inter-county arrangements for other services were borne in mind, in particular the regions for local government planning and development (in fact, only counties Roscommon and Meath are in different combinations with other counties for health purposes). Regard was also had to the desirability of not combining too many counties in any one board, of not allowing the population to be served to be much below 200,000 persons in any case and of not having any board covering too extensive an area. (As in the case of the boards of guardians, the convenience of members attending meetings was considered, with the car and train substituting for the horse as the way of travelling).

However, it was not by using any exact formula that the decision was taken to have eight boards. This result of the detailed discussions and consideration was necessarily a compromise based on commonsense rather than on science.

HEALTH BOARDS

Title of Board	Functional Area	Population (1971)	Membership							
			Local Authority Members	Medical Practitioners	Dentists	Pharmacists	General Nurses	Psychiatric Nurses	Ministerial Nominees	Total
Eastern Health Board	Dublin City and County, Counties Kildare and Wicklow (1,800 sq. miles)	987,000	19	9	1	1	1	1	3	35
Midland Health Board	Counties Laois, Longford, Offaly and Westmeath (2,250 sq. miles)	179,000	16	7	1	1	1	1	3	30
Mid-Western Health Board	Counties Clare, Limerick City and County, County Tipperary (N.R.) (3,040 sq. miles)	269,000	15	6	1	1	1	1	3	28
North-Eastern Health Board	Counties Cavan, Louth, Meath, Monaghan (1,950 sq. miles)	245,000	16	7	1	1	1	1	3	30
North-Western Health Board	Counties Donegal, Leitrim and Sligo (2,600 sq. miles)	187,000	14	6	1	1	1	1	3	27
South-Eastern Health Board	Counties Carlow, Kilkenny, Tipperary (S.R.), County and City of Waterford and County Wexford (6,630 sq. miles)	328,000	16	8	1	1	1	1	3	31
Southern Health Board	County and City of Cork and County Kerry (4,700 sq. miles)	465,000	18	8	1	1	1	1	3	33
Western Health Board	Counties Galway, Mayo and Roscommon (5,020 sq. miles)	311,000	15	7	1	1	1	1	3	29

The map opposite shows the functional areas of the boards.

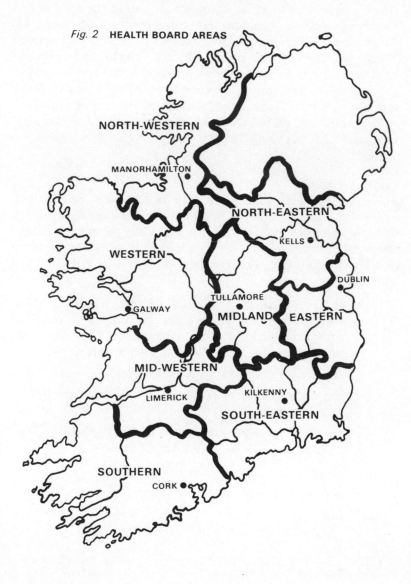

Fig. 2 **HEALTH BOARD AREAS**

Membership of health boards

Members of health boards come from many walks of life. An analysis of the occupations of the first members of the health boards, appointed in 1970, showed that, out of the total of 243 members, medical practitioners numbered 61, farmers 44, shopkeepers 33, nurses 17, pharmacists 10, dentists 8, teachers 7 and solicitors, trade union officials, clerks and company directors 6 each. Several other occupations are represented in the remaining appointees. People employed by a health board are not debarred from membership of it, except for those holding office as chief executive officer, programme manager, finance officer, personnel officer or planning and evaluation officer.[6]

Local committees

As required by section 7 of the 1970 Act, local committees, whose function is mainly advisory, have been established.[7] In the case of most counties, there is one local committee for the county. Local councillors are in a majority in the membership of these committees. The constitution for a county advisory committee is:

(i) three councillors from each electoral area (in those local authorities where there are only four electoral areas, the Council would appoint three further councillors to ensure a local authority majority),

(ii) the county manager (or his nominee),

(iii) the county medical officer (now the director of community care),

(iv) the resident medical superintendent of the district mental hospital (or a senior psychiatrist),

(v) a consultant from a general hospital,

(vi) two other doctors elected by the profession,

(vii) the superintendent assistance officer (now the superintendent community welfare officer),

[6]Rule 8 of Second Schedule, Health Act, 1970 and Health (Disqualification of Officers and Servants) Order, 1971.

[7]Under Section 7 of Health Act, 1970 and the Health (Local Committees) Regulations, 1972.

(viii) a psychiatric nurse,

 (ix) a public health nurse,

  (x) a dentist,

 (xi) a pharmacist,

(xii) two other persons, not being councillors, who are associated with voluntary organisations in the sphere of social services.

Meetings of a local committee are attended by the chief executive officer or another senior officer of the health board. This general pattern for the constitution of local committees is varied for the four areas which include county boroughs.

Management in health boards
Each health board is required to have 'a person who shall be called and shall act as the chief executive officer to the board'. The provisions in the 1970 Act on his functions make an interesting departure from those in the County Management Acts, which governed the management of the services under the former local administration. The Management Acts gave to the county manager the statutory responsibility for practically all the functions of the county council, although in performing them he was subject to restrictions and directions by the council. Under the 1970 Act only a limited range of decisions, mainly relating to eligibility of individuals for services and personnel matters, are reserved to the chief executive officer of a health board. Outside of these matters he and the other officers of the board are specifically required to 'act in accordance with such decisions and directions (whether of a general or a particular nature) as are conveyed to or through the chief executive officer by the board, and in accordance with any such decisions and directions so conveyed of a committee to which functions have been delegated by the board'. When the chief executive officer or another officer acts in accordance with such a direction, he is regarded as acting on behalf of the board.[8]

In fact, the health boards have recognised the need to delegate the day-to-day management of the services on a considerable scale to their chief executive officers, while retaining

[8]Section 17 of the Health Act, 1970.

ultimate control in their own hands. The following resolution is typical of those adopted by the boards:

'That the North Western Health Board, in accordance with Section 17(1) of the Health Act, 1970, hereby directs that the Chief Executive Officer shall, in the performance of his duties or in assigning duties or delegating functions to other officers, take such steps as are authorised by law and are necessary or desirable for the performance of the functions of the board otherwise than in relation to the following matters:

(a) the approval of estimates or of variations of estimates,

(b) the authorisation of capital schemes or the borrowing of money,

(c) the acquisition and disposal of land, or premises,

(d) decisions on programmes for development of services and review of such programmes,

(e) decisions under Section 38 of the Health Act, 1970, relating to the provision or discontinuance of premises,

and that the Chief Executive Officer may, to whatever extent he considers appropriate, delegate to other officers of the Board the performance of any of the duties and functions given to him under this direction, and that in carrying out this direction, the Chief Executive Officer shall comply with such instruction of a general nature as the Board may from time to time give to him, and that this direction may be revoked or amended by the Board at any time.'

The management team

The management consultants, Messrs. McKinsey and Co., who reported on the management processes and structure of the health boards, recommended that the work of the board be divided into three broad programmes, covering respectively community care services, general hospital services and 'special' hospital services (these being in the main the hospital services for the mentally ill and the mentally handicapped). Each of these programmes (the work under which is dealt with in later chapters) was to be put in charge of a 'programme manager'. In the larger boards, a separate programme manager for each of the three programmes was recommended while in each of the smaller boards (the Midland, Mid-Western, North-Eastern and North-Western Boards), there was provision for only two programme managers, one of whom covered the two hospital programmes.

In addition, the consultants recommended the appointment of 'functional' officers in charge of finance, personnel and planning (in the case of the smaller boards, finance and planning were combined under one officer). This group of officers, under the chief executive officer, form the 'management team' for the health board. The chart on page 57 illustrates the team for a large board.

Each member of the management team has his own specific responsibilities, but they are expected to act together as a group in evolving policy and advising the board on the future lines of development.

Each of the health boards adopted these management recommendations and, with the Minister's agreement, authorised the recruitment of the necessary staffs. The build-up of the management teams proceeded accordingly.

Fig. 3 **ORGANISATION IN A LARGER HEALTH BOARD AREA**

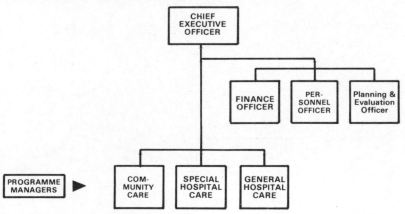

Community care staff

The community care programme of a health board covers the preventive health services, the general practitioner services, dental and public health nursing services and the field of activities of social workers. Direct administration of these services from the headquarters of the health board was not recommended; instead this programme is administered for a number of separate communities under each health board. The services in the community are co-ordinated by the director of community care.[9] He is responsible to the programme manager for the operation of this range of services within his community.

The recommended population to be served by each of these

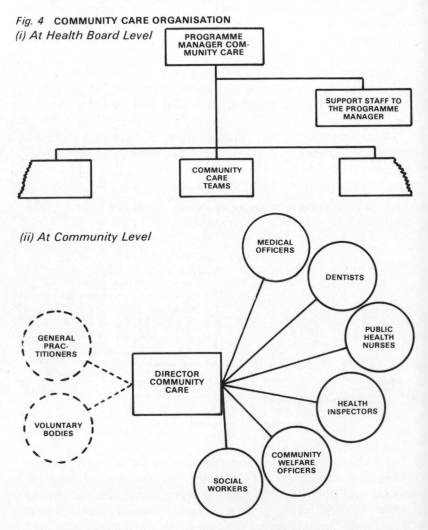

Fig. 4 **COMMUNITY CARE ORGANISATION**

(i) At Health Board Level

PROGRAMME MANAGER COMMUNITY CARE

SUPPORT STAFF TO THE PROGRAMME MANAGER

COMMUNITY CARE TEAMS

(ii) At Community Level

MEDICAL OFFICERS

DENTISTS

PUBLIC HEALTH NURSES

GENERAL PRACTITIONERS

DIRECTOR COMMUNITY CARE

HEALTH INSPECTORS

VOLUNTARY BODIES

COMMUNITY WELFARE OFFICERS

SOCIAL WORKERS

[9]The full title of this post, which is held by a doctor is 'director of community care and medical officer of health'.

communities is much the same as the population of the average county and, in practice, the county boundaries are usually accepted for the communities. In most areas, the first directors of community care were the former county medical officers.

The chart on page 58 illustrates the organisation of the community care programme. The positions on this chart do not necessarily indicate the relative status of the officers shown. The support staff and administrative staff shown for the programme manager and the director of community care would not, in most boards, be large in number.

Organisation for general hospitals

The programme manager, general hospital care, has responsibility for planning general hospital services for the population served by the health board. Unlike the programme manager for community care, he will not have under him a county or community organisation, but has a small support staff to assist him in his planning work.

It is intended that each of the major hospitals of a health board should have a competent resident hospital administrator and that smaller hospitals should be grouped for this purpose under one administrator. Health boards are also recommended to establish executive committees for the larger and more complex institutions, with membership and functions so designed as to draw the consultants and other staff in the hospital into its administration.

Special hospital programme staff

The main parts of the special hospital care programme are the care of psychiatric patients, geriatric services in hospitals, and the care of the mentally handicapped. Each health board took over a number of mental hospitals from the former local administration and these, of course, remain the centres from which the psychiatric services are organised. Under the programme manager, the officers directing the mental health service are the chief psychiatrists and, in larger urban areas, clinical directors for subdivisions of the area. Because the services for the mentally handicapped are provided mainly in voluntary institutions, most health boards have no special directorate for this service.

Other Executive Bodies

Not all the executive work in relation to the health services is suited to local administration. For those parts of it not so suited, the practice evolved of setting up special central executive agencies. Some of these were set up by special statutes and others were formerly set up by arranging for the establishment of a company under the Companies Acts. Among the former, the most noteworthy example is probably the Voluntary Health Insurance Board; the latter included the Medical Research Council and bodies to administer the blood transfusion service and the mass radiography service.

The Health (Corporate Bodies) Act, 1961 brought in a new, more easily used procedure for setting up such executive bodies. The Minister is authorised to set up a corporate body to administer a health service by an order under the Act. Such an order, which is liable to annulment by either House of the Oireachtas, specifies the constitution and functions of the body established and includes provision on the appointment of staff, etc. This Act has been used to set up many new executive agencies, including the Medico-Social Research Board, the National Drugs Advisory Board, the Hospitals Joint Services Board and the Health Education Bureau.

A provision of the 1961 Act allowed the limited liability companies established earlier as executive bodies for the health services to become transformed into bodies under the new Act by passing a simple resolution. This provision has been used by a number of those companies. The Blood Transfusion Service Board and the National Rehabilitation Board are among the bodies which were so transformed. A full list of the executive bodies set up under the 1961 Act and of the other executive bodies is contained in Appendix A.

There is power to authorise the health boards (or two or more of them) to act through a specially established joint board.[10] The first use of this provision for joint action of health boards arose in the administration of a central bureau for paying doctors and chemists under the re-organised general medical service described in Chapter 10. The body concerned

[10]Section 11 of the Health Act, 1970.

with this is the General Medical Services (Payments) Board.

While the voluntary hospitals are not, of course, executive bodies within the sphere of public administration, like those referred to above, an account of the executive agencies in the health services would be incomplete without referring to those hospitals. They are usually the property of the religious orders and voluntary bodies who are charged with their administration. The voluntary hospitals participate in a large way in providing services for the public authorities. As well as the voluntary hospitals there are a number of other associations and agencies which co-operate with the public authorities in the provision of the health services. Included among these are councils or associations for specific diseases or conditions and bodies concerned in the organisation of social services.

International Health Organisations

Ireland plays its part in a number of inter-governmental health bodies and its services benefit from participation in the work of these bodies through information obtained on what is done elsewhere, through reports of international technical work and through sending her own nationals abroad on study tours organised by these bodies.

The World Health Organisation
The World Health Organisation (WHO) is paramount among the international health bodies. This Organisation was founded in 1948 as a specialised agency of the United Nations Organisation and took over the work of the International Office of Public Health of the League of Nations. The Constitution of the Organisation[11] lists its functions, the more important and general ones being: to act as the directing and co-ordinating authority on international health work; to assist Governments, upon request, in strengthening health services and to furnish technical assistance and in emergencies, necessary aid.

The legislative organ of WHO is the annual assembly. This is attended by representatives of the 149 member states of the Organisation. At the assembly, the budget is approved, international regulations are made and questions of general interest

[11]This, and other publications of the Organisation may be purchased through the Government Publications Sale Office, G.P.O. Arcade, Dublin.

are debated. The responsibility for seeing that the decisions of the Assembly are carried out is vested in the Executive Board of the Organisation which is made up of persons nominated by thirty member states. The staff of WHO is headed by a Director-General. It is his responsibility to propose the budget for submission by the Executive Board to the Assembly and to see to the execution of the decisions of the Assembly and the Board. The headquarters of the Organisation is in Geneva. Its total budget for 1978 was about £95 million, of which Ireland contributed about £228,000.

The execution of the policies of WHO is to a great extent delegated to subsidiary regional organisations, that with which this country is concerned being the European Regional Office, with headquarters in Copenhagen. The regional organisations have their own staffs and work in conjunction with regional committees comprising representatives of the member states of the region.

The Organisation has power to make regulations binding on its members. The most important of these are the International Sanitary Regulations which govern the restrictions which may be imposed on the movements of international traffic to prevent the spread of infectious diseases,[12] and the International Regulations on Health Statistics which provide a standardised list of diseases and causes of death.[13]

The benefit derived by the more highly-developed members of WHO comes through fellowships and seminars organised by the regional organisations. A number of fellowships are granted each year to each member of the region and the individual states are accorded a wide discretion in choosing the fellows and the subjects of study. The arrangements for the course of study in each case are made by the Organisation, whose wide experience is very valuable in this respect. A wide variety of studies has been pursued by Irish fellows under this scheme.

The Council of Europe
The Council of Europe is an organisation of twenty European States (Austria, Belgium, Cyprus, Denmark, France, the Federal Republic of Germany, Greece, Iceland, Ireland, Italy, Luxembourg,

[12]See Chapter Ten.
[13]See Chapter Thirteen.

Malta, Netherlands, Norway, Portugal, Spain, Sweden, Switzerland, Turkey and the United Kingdom), which was established in 1949. Its aim is 'to achieve a greater unity between its members for the purpose of safeguarding and realising the ideals and principles which are their common heritage and facilitating their economic and social progress'. Health questions are not, of course, the primary concern of the Council of Europe but its programme includes the encouragement of its members to co-operate with each other in providing health services and to co-ordinate their health programmes. In this it aims not to duplicate the work of WHO, with which it maintains liaison. Representatives of the health administrations of the member states of the Council meet twice yearly in Strasbourg. Among steps towards co-ordination are the establishment of direct contacts between the administrations and examination of the technical and administrative difficulties in the way of mutual aid in providing health services, both normally and in times of disasters. The Council also provides fellowships for members of the medical and 'paramedical' professions and of the health services to become conversant with new techniques practised in European countries and to participate in studies and research of common European interest. Several of these fellowships have been awarded to candidates from Ireland.

Eleven of the member states of the Council of Europe—Austria, Belgium, Denmark, France, Federal Republic of Germany, Ireland, Italy, Luxembourg, the Netherlands, Switzerland and the United Kingdom—have, under the aegis of the Council, entered into a 'partial agreement' to co-operate in certain public health matters. They deal in particular with arrangements for health control of sea and air travel, with health controls on foodstuffs and with controls on poisonous substances in agriculture. The Committee set up under this 'partial agreement' meets regularly in Strasbourg and in other European centres.

The European Communities
These are the European Economic Community (The EEC or Common Market), set up in 1958 under the Treaty of Rome, the European Atomic Energy Agency and the European Coal and Steel Community. The present members of the Com-

munities are Belgium, Denmark, France, Federal Republic of Germany, Ireland, Italy, Luxembourg, the Netherlands and the United Kingdom. While the Treaty of Rome, under which the main community—the European Economic Community—was set up contains little specific provisions on health services, the activities of the Communities include a number of matters relating to the health services and these involve certain obligations for this country.

It is an aim of the Treaty of Rome to allow nationals of each of the member states of the EEC freedom to work in other member states and the Commission of the Community has the duty to issue directives to bring this freedom about. These directives include requirements for mutual recognition of professional qualifications and registrations between the member states. Directives have already been made for doctors and nurses and draft directives for dentists, midwives, pharmacists and opticians are at present being examined. These directives are referred to again on page 84. ·

Also in furtherance of the aim of having free movement of workers, the European Economic Community has made regulations[14] for migrant workers, so that they can carry entitlement to social services from one country to another, both for themselves and their dependants. This involves our health administration in obligations to arrange health services for workers from other countries in the Community who are temporarily in Ireland and liability will have to be assumed for health care of eligible Irish workers who are temporarily in one of those countries.

Other regulations of the European Economic Community designed to remove causes of distortion in competition, are designed to introduce standardisation in the controls on the manufacture and sale of a number of products. The Department of Health is involved in this respect as far as quality control of pharmaceutical products and the Regulations governing additives and colouring matters in food are concerned.

As well as this involvement in the operation and subsequent evolution of these controls, it is clear that, because of the wide scope of the European Communities and the nature of obligations attached to membership, our health administration will be

---

[14]It will be seen from the 1978 Estimates that a payment of £3,300,000 to this country is budgeted for under these regulations.

increasingly involved in many activities arising from membership. Meetings of the Ministers for Health of the nine member countries took place in December, 1977 and December, 1978.

Entry into the Communities has affected our health services in a number of ways, but there is nothing in the Treaty of Rome or in the activities of the Community up to the present which would suggest that a common health care system will become obligatory for the members.

Other inter-Governmental organisations
Some other organisations representative of their member states are concerned with health questions and the Irish health services benefit from their activities. The United Nations Organisation (UNO) itself is responsible for the administration of the conventions on traffic in dangerous drugs; another of its specialised agencies, the Food and Agriculture Organisation (FAO), has functions in connection with nutrition and food standards; and the International Labour Office (ILO) concerns itself with such matters as standards for social security (including eligibility for health services), medical examination of various classes of workers and the rehabilitation of the disabled. The International Civil Aviation Organisation (ICAO) which regulates international air traffic, is concerned with the extent of the health precautions required for such traffic under WHO regulations. The International Atomic Energy Agency deals with health protection in the field of nuclear energy.

Other international bodies
As well as the bodies representative of Governments, there are a large number of international health organisations which are directly representative of professional or specialised interests in countries throughout the world. The World Medical Association (WMA), for example, is representative of the medical associations of most countries. In addition to organising its own meetings at which professional subjects are discussed, the Association holds a watching brief on behalf of the medical profession at the Assemblies of WHO. The International Hospital Federation is another example of these bodies. Its members are bodies interested in hospital construction and administration.

Chapter Six

Personnel

The health services are concerned with the provision of services by persons for persons. The 'health care industry' is, therefore, highly labour intensive. It employs over 54,000 people—that is, about 5·2 per cent of the total workforce—and there are over 300 different grades of staff. Annual expenditure on staff in 1977 was in the region of £200 million or about 60 per cent of current public expenditure on the health services.

Employment in Health Boards etc.

Numbers employed
Understandably the eight health boards are the biggest employers. However, large numbers of personnel are also employed by other health agencies which are wholly or mainly financed by the State, mainly the voluntary hospitals, the homes for the mentally handicapped and a number of specialist bodies. The following is a breakdown of the number of posts on 31 December, 1977:

Table 1—Employment in Health Boards, etc.

Agency	Posts
Health boards	33,038
Voluntary and other public hospitals	16,417
Homes for the mentally handicapped	3,195
Other health bodies	1,400
Total	54,050

The health boards and the public hospitals employ almost 92 per cent of all those working in the health services—49,455 posts in all. The distribution of these 49,455 posts between the main categories was as follows:

Table 2—Health board and public hospital posts

Category	Posts
Medical and dental	3,215
Nursing	28,190
Paramedical	2,090
Catering/housekeeping	7,170
Maintenance	2,350
Administrative	4,460
Other	1,980
Total	49,455

The percentage distribution of staff between the major health care programmes is:

Table 3—Staff distribution between health care programme

Programme	Percentage
General hospital care (including obstetrics)	
Special hospital care (psychiatry, mental handicap, physical handicap, infectious diseases, long-stay etc.)	43
	28
Community care (general medical services, home nursing, public health, preventive services, etc.)	24
Support services	5
Total	100

For some purposes, the health boards, instead of employing officers and servants, make agreements with individuals to provide the services on a contract basis. The service in which this has been done on the biggest scale is the general medical service which is discussed in Chapter 10. The percentages shown above do not, therefore relate to all those actually working in the different programmes.

Personnel policy

The importance of effective personnel policy in relation to the satisfactory functioning of the health services is being increasingly recognised at all levels. This has been reflected both at health board and national levels. At health board level there is a separate personnel function for each board, while in the recent restructuring of the Department of Health special attention was paid to the personnel function and a new personnel unit was created to deal with personnel issues at a national level. The other health agencies, such as the voluntary hospitals, and other voluntary organisations also play a vital role both in the management of their own personnel and in assisting in the formulation of national policies for the various grades and types of staff.

Having regard to the number and variety of grades the task confronting the personnel managers in the health service is undoubtedly a formidable one. The broad aim is to anticipate as far as possible the requirements of the services and the reasonable needs of the various staff categories rather than react to pressures which might build up. This has to be achieved on the following fronts:

— recruitment;
— staff training and development;
— remuneration and conditions of service;
— formulation, implementation and monitoring of personnel policies in relation to specific related staff groups;
— liaison with the EEC in directives for mutual recognition of qualifications, etc.

Recruitment and Employment of staff

Chapter II of Part II of the Health Act, 1970, provides a code governing the appointment and employment of personnel in health boards. The determination of the number and kinds of officers and servants to be appointed is made by the board in accordance with the directions of the Minister. The making of appointments, and the determination of remuneration and conditions of employment are, however, reserved to the chief executive officer of the board and he, in taking decisions on these, must act in accordance with the directions of the Minister.

These directions are quite detailed and are set out in Appendix B.

For the more senior classes of officer (including many of the professional posts) selection is made through the Local Appointments Commissioners. In other cases selection is made through the chief executive officer in accordance with a selection procedure specified by the Minister. Qualifications for the various classes of officer under the health boards are determined by the Minister.[1] There is an age limit—normally sixty-five years—for employment.

Officers of health boards may be either permanent or temporary. The latter are appointed for a fixed term and the former have security of tenure, but may be suspended or removed from office by the chief executive officer following a procedure laid down in the Act. This involves investigation of the cause put forward for removal by a special committee with a chairman appointed by the Minister and an even number of other persons, of whom half are staff representatives and the other half are selected from a panel nominated by the chief executive officer.

The voluntary hospitals and other agencies are responsible for the selection of their own staff. However, qualifications for those appointed and conditions of employment are substantially the same for similar grades of personnel whether employed by health boards or other health agencies.

Like their fellow employees in other employments, health staffs are covered by the many reforms which have taken place in the employment field in recent years. Of these, the removal of the marriage bar in the public service and the Employment Equality Act, 1977 are particularly significant for the health services.

In the case of consultant medical staff, Comhairle na nOspidéal plays an important role. It regulates the numbers and types of consultant appointments in hospitals providing services under the Health Acts and specifies professional qualifications for appointments.

The Health Act, 1970 also empowered the Minister to make regulations giving the Comhairle functions in the selection of

[1] In the case of medical consultants, the professional qualifications are specified by Comhairle na nOispidéal.

consultants for health board and voluntary hospitals. At the Minister's request, the Comhairle has prepared a scheme for a common selection procedure. At the time of writing, this is being discussed between the Department of Health and the various representative interests concerned. The 1970 Act requires that, before regulations on a common selection procedure are executed a draft of them must be submitted for approval to the Dáil and Seanad.

Remuneration and Conditions of Service
Nearly all categories of health boards staffs are covered by a conciliation and arbitration scheme for health boards and local authorities. There is a national body—the Local Government Staff Negotiations Board—to represent management in the operation of this scheme. The Department of Health and the chief executive officers of the health boards are represented on it. Responsibility for the overall operation of the scheme is vested in a National Joint Council which consists of an equal number of members of the Board and of the 'staff panel' (comprised of appropriate staff associations), under the chairmanship of an officer of the Labour Court.

Some health board staff (notably psychiatric nurses and the non-officer grades) have access to the Labour Court. All staff employed by voluntary hospitals and other health bodies have access to the Labour Court.

Permanent staff of health boards have the same superannuation scheme as those in local authorities. It is a contributory scheme and provides for lump sum payments and pensions on retirement. There is also a contributory widows and orphans pension scheme for male staff. Salaried staffs in voluntary hospitals have similar arrangements for superannuation.

Continuing Education and Training
The Council for Post-Graduate Medical and Dental Education which was established in 1973 has responsibility for postgraduate education and training of doctors and dentists. Provision has been made in the Medical Practitioners Act, 1978, for the taking over of its functions by a statutory body to be known as the Post-Graduate Medical and Dental Board. These are:
(a) to promote the development of post-graduate medical and

dental education and training and to co-ordinate such developments;

(b) to advise the Minister, after consultation with such other bodies as the Board may consider appropriate, on all matters, including financial matters, relating to the development and co-ordination of post-graduate medical and dental training;

(c) whenever appropriate, to organise post-graduate education and training for registered medical practitioners and registered dentists;

(d) to provide career guidance for registered medical practitioners and registered dentists, and

(e) such other function as may be assigned to it from time to time by the Minister.

Health boards and voluntary hospitals have over the past number of years made an increased investment in terms of money, time and effort in continuing staff development. They are involved in and participate in the basic training of many health professions. In 1978, for example, they budgeted to spend over £350,000 on specialised training courses for staff development and in meeting or contributing towards post-graduate education and training courses for their staffs.

Most of the money spent by health agencies on specialised training is devoted to the post-graduate training schemes provided by bodies such as Faculties of the Medical Schools, clinical societies, medical associations, university departments and to some extent private bodies. In addition, staff undergoing examinations for higher degrees or diplomas are granted special leave with pay, and in the case of whole-time medical, dental and nursing staffs a fortnight's study leave with pay prior to examination is usually granted. An Bord Altranais, in addition to providing post qualification training for nurses, co-ordinates the activities of other bodies engaged in the area of training for nurses.

The Council of the Pharmaceutical Society is the governing body for pharmaceutical chemists. It lays down the training programme which is a combination of theoretical and practical instruction with apprenticeship under a member of the society. Training facilities are available for paramedical groups such as physiotherapists, radiographers, medical laboratory technicians, health inspectors and occupational therapists and these lead to recognised qualifications which are required for persons employed in our health service.

As regards clerical and administrative staffs, induction training is normally provided by the individual employing health agency. Health agencies usually avail of the courses provided by 'outside' training and educational institutions to enable their staffs to acquire further interpersonal and management skills. In this area, the Institute of Public Administration is the largest training agency, whilst staff also attend courses run by the Institute of Hospital Administrators, School of Management Studies, Rathmines and the Irish Management Institute.

The facilities usually granted to staff attending short training courses are special leave with pay together with recoupment of the course fee and appropriate travelling and subsistence expenses.

Where recruitment difficulties exist, health agencies become involved in sponsorship arrangements for trainee health personnel, particularly in the paramedical area. Such students are usually paid a grant towards their fees by health boards in response for an undertaking that the trainee will work for a specified period on qualification with the sponsoring agency. In 1976, for example, over a hundred student physiotherapists, occupational therapists, speech therapists and medical laboratory technicians were sponsored in this way.

The Health Staff Development Committee, which is representative of the Department of Health, the health boards, the voluntary hospitals, An Bord Altranais and the Institute of Public Administration, was established in 1971. Its main functions are the preparation of the annual programme of post-recruitment management and skills training for health personnel and the consequent evaluation and review of these programmes.

Medical Practitioners

Medical practitioners in Ireland and Great Britain were first registered under the Medical Act of 1858 and a separate Irish register was founded in 1927, when the Medical Registration Council was set up. The bodies whose qualifying diplomas are now recognised are the National University of Ireland, the University of Dublin and the Royal Colleges of Physicians and Surgeons.

At the time of writing, the Medical Registration Council is still in existence and the 1927 Act is extant. However, a comprehensive new statute—the Medical Practitioners Act, 1978—will shortly come into effect. This will replace the Medical Registration Council with a new Medical Council. The other provisions of the 1927 Act will also be replaced. The following paragraphs are based on a projection to the time when the new Act will be in full operation.

The Medical Council[2]
There will be twenty-five members including its President, on the Medical Council. It will be constituted of four persons appointed by the Minister, ten members elected by registered medical practitioners, five members by the undergraduate schools and six members appointed by the appropriate postgraduate bodies. The Council will have a term of office of five years. It will be financed entirely from registration fees. Its principal functions will be:

(a) the general registration of all medical practitioners and also the registration of specialist doctors,
(b) responsibility for standards of education and training at both undergraduate and post-graduate levels,
(c) all matters relating to fitness to practise, and
(d) certain designated functions in relation to the operation and implementation of the EEC doctors' directives, such as enquiries from other Member States relating to the character or health and the verification of qualifications of Irish registered doctors moving to another Member State.

Medical Registration
The most important duty of the Medical Council will be to keep the General Register of Medical Practitioners. Each student obtaining any of the approved primary qualifications[3] is entitled

---

[2] See sections 6 to 25 of the 1978 Act.
[3] They are listed in the Fourth Schedule to the 1978 Act.

to be provisionally registered and then, after completing a year's internship, may become fully registered. A national of a member state of the European Economic Community who has been awarded a qualification in medicine by the competent authority in his native country is entitled to be registered in the Irish Register; Irish nationals are entitled to be included in the Registers of other Member States on a similar basis. A national of a non-EEC country may also be granted registration if the Medical Council is satisfied that he has obtained a qualification in medicine of an appropriate standard.

Effect of Registration
Registered medical practitioners are qualified by law to sign medical certificates[4] and prescribe certain dangerous drugs.[5] Outside of doing these things, an unregistered person may give medical treatment but would be liable to penalties if he represents himself as being registered. Furthermore, he would not be entitled to sue for fees and he would not be eligible for any public appointment.[6]

Temporary Registration
Doctors from a number of foreign states, after qualification, are employed in Irish hospitals to gain experience. To facilitate this practice by removing from these residents the disabilities referred to in the preceding paragraph a system of temporary registration is provided for.[7] This permits the Council to register any foreign graduate whose qualifications it regards as adequate. Temporary registration is limited to whatever period the Council fixes in each case and lapses in any event when the foreign graduate is no longer employed in the hospital. The aggregate of periods of temporary registration which the Council is empowered to grant may not exceed five years.

Specialist Registration
Under section 30 of the 1978 Act the Medical Council is empowered, but not obliged, with the consent of the Minister, to prepare and establish a register of medical specialists. This will

4Section 59 of 1978 Act.
5See Chapter 10.
6Section 60 of 1978 Act.
7Section 29 of 1978 Act.

enable this country, should it be so decided, to follow the practice which exists in most continental countries (but not in the United Kingdom).

Medical Training Standards

The Medical Council will have the duty of satisfying itself that the standard of knowledge required at examinations held by the medical schools is adequate.[8] In the event of the Council deciding that a medical school was no longer adequate there is a procedure whereby the Minister on the recommendation of the Council can withdraw recognition. The Council also must satisfy itself that clinical training and experience provided during the 'intern year' is of an appropriate standard. It also has the duty to ensure that standards of post-graduate education and training provided by bodies recognised by it for medical specialist training are adequate and for ensuring that minimum EEC requirements in this regard are met.

Numbers registered

The Medical Register for 1977 shows that on 31 December 1976 there were 10,953 fully registered medical practitioners. This total included many not practising in the country. In the 1971 census of population 3,565 residents of the State were returned as medical practitioners, against 9,642 registered medical practitioners in December 1971.

Dentists

The law on the control of the dental profession is closely related to that on medical practitioners and was affected similarly by the establishment of the Irish Free State in the nineteen-twenties.

The Dental Board[9]

The Dental Board, which was established under the Dentists Act, 1928, has a membership of nine, made up of one Government nominee, three nominated by the Medical Registration

[8]Section 35 of 1978 Act.
[9]Sections 3 to 21 of and Second Schedule to Dentists Act, 1928.

Council and five dentists elected by dentists resident in the State. The members' term of office is five years. The Board's expenses are met from fees for registration and for retention on the register.

The functions of the Dental Board and the Medical Registration Council
The Dental Board partners the Medical Registration Council (and its successor the Medical Council) in the regulation of the dental profession. The Board's primary duty is to keep the Register of Dentists, while the Council is charged with the surveillance of the qualifying examinations for dentists and has for that purpose powers similar to those which it has for medical examinations. When acting in relation to a dental school, the Council has three additional members who are dentists appointed by the Board. The bodies granting degrees in dentistry are the National University of Ireland, the University of Dublin and the Royal College of Surgeons. The period of training is six years.

Registration[10]
Those passing the recognised qualifying examinations are entitled to be registered on paying the requisite fee (there is no provisional registration for dentists). The provisions for registration of British-trained dentists here and Irish-trained dentists in Britain are similar to those for medical practitioners. Reciprocity with other foreign States is also provided for but the making of any reciprocity agreement does not seem to have arisen.

Practice of dentistry
Unregistered persons may not practise dentistry.[11] Only registered dentists, registered medical practitioners and, in certain emergency conditions, chemists are permitted to extract teeth. Other parts of the practice of dentistry are reserved to dentists and medical practitioners but mechanics and their apprentices may be employed in dental workshops. The repair of dentures, without fitting them, is not controlled. With certain

[10]Sections 26 to 30 of 1928 Act.
[11]Section 45 of 1928 Act.

exceptions, bodies corporate (such as limited liability companies) may not engage in the practice of dentistry.[12]

Number of dentists

There were 864 names on the Dental Register on 1 January, 1976. As dentists, unlike medical practitioners, must pay retention fees annually to have their names kept on the register, this figure is probably close to that for the number of practising dentists. In the 1971 Census returns 659 persons showed dentistry as their occupation, as opposed to 785 names on the Dental Register on 1 January 1972.

Nurses and Midwives

An Bord Altranais

There are more in the nursing profession than in any of the other health professions and nurses are divided into several categories. The body controlling them is an Bord Altranais which has twentythree members. Twelve are nurses representing the different branches of the profession, seven are medical practitioners and the rest are representative of health boards, educational authorities and other interests. Ten of the nurses are elected by those on the nurses' register: the other members are appointed by the Minister for Health, but in making most of the appointments he is required to consult with representative organisations.[13] The Board controls both nurses and midwives ('nurse' in the Nurses Act, 1950, is defined as including a midwife). It has a special Midwives Committee, made up of some of the board members and some others to deal particularly with disciplinary matters affecting midwives.[14] The term of office of members of An Bord Altranais and the Midwives Committee is five years. The Minister for Health appoints the President of the Board.

The Board's expenses are met mainly from the examination and registration fees paid by the nurses and from fees paid by participants in courses run by the Board. Grants towards the

[12]Section 46 of 1928 Act.
[13]The detailed constitution of An Bord Altranais is given in Sections 12 and 13 of the Nurses Act, 1950.
[14]See Sections 29 to 38 of the Act of 1950.

expenses of the Board may be made by the Minister for Health. The Minister's controlling functions in relation to the Board exceed those he has in the cases of the Medical Registration Council and the Dental Board.

Registration of nurses and midwives[15]

An Bord Altranais keeps a Register of Nurses with separate divisions for general trained nurses (entitled to use the initials R.G.N.), mental handicap nurses (R.N.M.H.), midwives (R.M.), psychiatric nurses (R.P.N.) and sick children's nurses (R.S.C.N.). The persons entitled to be registered are those who have taken the course of training prescribed by the Board and passed its examinations or who have an equivalent nursing qualification obtained outside the State. There are also supplementary divisions of the register for orthopaedic nurses, public health nurses, tuberculosis nurses and for tutors.

Training of nurses and midwives[16]

The Board has, in relation to the training of nurses and midwives, powers more direct and detailed than those which the Medical Council and the Dental Board have as respects their professions. The detailed syllabus for training is laid down by the Board and the training hospitals must be approved by the Board and must comply with its conditions for recognition.[17] These conditions include provisions as to the size of the hospital, the teaching staff and the accommodation and facilities available to the student nurses. There are some 75 recognised training hospitals in the country, of which 29 are for training general nurses, 24 for psychiatric nurses, 10 for midwives, 8 for mental handicap nurses, 3 for sick children's nurses and one for orthopaedic nurses.

The period of training for general, psychiatric, sick children's and mental handicap nursing is three years and for the midwives division of the register one year. The combined periods are contracted in the case of a nurse studying for registration in a second division of the Register.

The Board has power itself to participate in the actual train-

---

[15]Sections 41 to 49 of the Act of 1950 and the Nurses Rules, 1953 (the latter are published by the Board).

[16]Sections 50 to 55 of Act of 1950.

[17]The Board publishes a list of minimum standards for nurse training schools. This is obtainable from the Board.

ing of nurses. In general, it does not do this for student nurses but it has equipped premises in which special training courses are given for registered nurses. In particular, it has organised post-graduate courses of training in public health nursing. The Board itself appoints examiners and conducts the qualifying examinations for nurses. The examinations are held in training hospitals throughout the country.

Effect of registration
Registration as a nurse entitles one to use the title of registered nurse and it is an offence for anyone who is not registered to do so or to give the impression that she (or he) is registered.[18] There is, however, no prohibition on anyone practising nursing. This is not so in the case of midwifery. Attendance on women in childbirth is restricted by law, except where urgency makes this impracticable, to registered midwives and medical practitioners (and to *bona fide* students for these professions).[19]

Practice of midwifery
Midwives in practising their profession are required to comply with detailed rules laid down by the Board.[20] They are supervised in their work by the health boards.[21]

Numbers of nurses and midwives
The number of registered nurses in each category on 31 December 1977 are detailed below

Table 4—Registered nurses by category

Category	Number
General nurses	41,603
Psychiatric nurses	12,699
Midwives	20,414
Sick childrens' nurses	2,033
Infectious diseases nurses	1,809
Mental handicap nurses	754
Orthopaedic nurses	68

[18]Section 56 of Act of 1950.
[19]Section 48 of the Midwives Act, 1944.
[20]Rules of Practice for Midwives-published by the Board.
[21]Sections 33 to 37 of Act of 1944.

As several nurses are registered in more than one division of the Register and as many of those registered have ceased to practise, these figures are not those of the nurses employed in this country. In the 1971 Census of Population, 19,284 persons returned their occupation as nursing (this includes mental nurses and trainee nurses).

Pharmaceutical Chemists

The origin of pharmaceutical chemists and their ancillaries as we now know them is best described in the preamble to the Pharmacy Act, 1875—one of those informative nineteenth century preambles which the development of the science of legal drafting has, rather unfortunately, cut out of modern Acts of Parliament. It is worth citing fairly fully:

'Whereas by an Act passed by the Parliament of Ireland in the thirty-first year of the reign of His Majesty George the Third ... it is enacted that no person shall open shop or practice the art and mystery of an apothecary within the kingdom of Ireland until he shall have been examined as to his qualifications and knowledge of the business by the persons and in the manner by the said Act prescribed, and shall have received a certificate to open shop or follow the art and mystery of an apothecary within the kingdom of Ireland from the Governor and Directors of the Apothecaries' Hall of the City of Dublin:

And whereas a great deficiency exists throughout Ireland of establishments and shops for the sale of medicines and compounding of prescriptions, and great inconvenience thereby arises to the public in many parts of the country:

And whereas to remedy such inconvenience it is expedient to amend the Act of 1791, and to enable persons who, although they do not desire to practise the art and mystery of an apothecary, desire and are qualified to open shop for the retailing dispensing and compounding of poisons and medical prescriptions, to keep open shop for the purposes aforesaid:

And whereas for the purposes aforesaid, it is expedient that provisions ... should be made for the formation of a

Pharmaceutical Society in Ireland . . .'

Thus was born the profession of pharmaceutical chemist as it is known to-day.

The Pharmaceutical Society of Ireland[22]

The Council of the Pharmaceutical Society, which is the governing body for pharmaceutical chemists, has twenty-one members who are elected by the members of the Society. Anyone who qualifies as a pharmaceutical chemist is entitled to be a member as long as he continues to pay the annual fees required. Those who do not pay the annual membership subscriptions are licentiates of the Society. These pay annual fees at a lower rate and have the same rights as members in the practice of pharmacy but have no say in the election of the Council. One third of the members of the Council go out of office each year. Registration fees, membership subscriptions and fees from students for the Society's courses finance its activities.

Registration of pharmaceutical chemists, etc.

Anyone who has completed the Society's prescribed course of training is entitled to registration as a pharmaceutical chemist.[23] Some lesser grades qualified to perform only part of the work of a pharmacist (in particular registered druggists) were created by the Pharmacy Acts but the only one of these now open to entrants is the grade of Assistant. A separate Register of Assistants is kept.

Training of pharmaceutical chemists

The training of pharmaceutical chemists is a combination of theoretical and practical instruction with apprenticeship under a member of the Society. The student wishing to become a pharmaceutical chemist must complete a four-year course of studies leading to the Degree of Bachelor of Science (Pharmacy). This is followed by a one-year apprenticeship in an approved pharmacy at the end of which it is necessary to pass an examination in forensic pharmacy. He then becomes eligible for registration as pharmaceutical chemist. Phar-

[22]Sections 4 to 18 of Pharmacy (Ireland) Act, 1875.
[23]Section 22 of 1875 Act.

maceutical assistants must complete a three-year apprenticeship with a pharmaceutical chemist followed by a part-time
course of lectures and practicals lasting about six months.[24]

Privileges attached to registration

Only those registered by the Society are permitted to 'keep
open shop for retailing, dispensing or compounding poisons . . .
or medical prescriptions'.[25] Pharmaceutical chemists also have
a special status and responsibilities in dealing in dangerous narcotic drugs and certain other drugs which may be sold only on
a medical or similar prescription.[26]

Numbers of pharmaceutical chemists

There were 1994 pharmaceutical chemists on the register on 1
January 1977. In addition, there were 611 assistants, 31
registered druggists and 23 dispensing chemists and druggists
(a grade with practically all the rights but not title of pharmaceutical chemist). The 1971 Census of Population indicated
that there were then 1,232 proprietors of chemists' businesses
and 1,571 employees in such business.

Opticians

Bord na Radharcmhastóirí[27]

Bord na Radharcmhastóirí (The Opticians Board) was set up
under the Opticians Act, 1956, to arrange for registration of
opticians and to supervise them in the practice of their profession. The Board has eleven members made up of four registered
medical practitioners, six opticians and one other person. The
term of office of Board members is five years. Its expenses are
met from examination and registration fees and fees for courses
of instruction given by it.

Registration of opticians [28]

The Board maintains two registers, one for ophthalmic opti-

---

[24]The Regulations on the courses and examinations for pharmacists are published
by the Society.
[25]Section 30 of 1875 Act.
[26]See page 207.
[27]Sections 5 to 22 of Opticians Act, 1956.
[28]Sections 23 to 41 of the 1956 Act.

cians (who both prescribe and supply spectacles) and one for dispensing opticians (who only supply spectacles on the prescription of others). Those who undergo the courses of training and who pass the examinations prescribed by the Board are registered. The Board may also register foreign-trained opticians.

Training and examinations [29]
The Board may itself provide training or may approve of other bodies to train opticians. Similarly, the Board may conduct the examinations or may appoint other bodies to do so under the Board's rules. Post-registration courses for opticians may be provided.

Prescription and sale of spectacles [30]
The prescription of spectacles is confined to registered medical practitioners and ophthalmic opticians and dispensing of prescriptions is limited to these and to dispensing opticians. The sale of spectacles by unqualified persons is prohibited. Opticians, for their part, are restricted by law in their practice to the provision of spectacles and, in the case of ophthalmic opticians, their prescription. An optician is specifically prohibited from treating eye disease, or from prescribing or administering drugs for that purpose or to paralyse the accommodation of the eye, and from suggesting that he is capable of making a medical diagnosis of eye disease.

The Board has made rules to regulate and control opticians in their practice and to control advertising by opticians. The titles of ophthalmic optician and dispensing optician are protected by the Act.

Numbers of opticians
On 31 December 1977, there were 223 registered ophthalmic opticians and 250 registered dispensing opticians. Not all of these are in wholetime practice as opticians.

[29]Sections 42 to 46 of the 1956 Act.
[30]Sections 47 to 53 of the 1956 Act.

Other personnel

The above descriptions have been confined to the professional categories for which there is statutory registration. There are, of course, many other important groups contributing to the services. These include such medical auxiliaries as physiotherapists, radiographers, chiropodists, dieticians and laboratory technicians and other groups such as the health inspectors and those working in social fields concerned with the health services. While these are not given statutory registration, there is a recognised qualification required in each case for persons employed in the services.

Finally, there is the corps of administrative staff, the top echelons of which are mentioned in Chapter Five. A series of grades for this staff has been evolved, with a system of job evaluation, so that a career structure, with promotional ladders, is provided within the health boards.

EEC Directives

Part of the provisions of the Treaty of Rome relating to the abolition of restrictions on the freedom of nationals of member states to provide services in the territory of the other member states is concerned with the mutual recognition of qualifications and diplomas in the professions. The mutual recognition of medical qualifications and freedom of movement of doctors within the EEC were the subject of the first directives adopted in 1975 by the Council of the European Community in respect of professional groups in the Member States. They came into effect in all member states in December 1976. Similar directives in relation to nurses were adopted in June 1977 and will come into operation in June 1979 and directives for dentists were adopted in July 1978, to come into effect early in 1980. Draft directives for midwives and opticians are at the time of writing under examination by expert working parties representative of the nine Member States.

Chapter Seven

Finance

Health expenditure is customarily divided into non-capital and capital categories. These categories are not water-tight as expenditure on repairs and replacements met from current revenue is not always easily distinguishable from purely capital expenditure. With these reservations, the two types of expenditure are dealt with separately in this Chapter.

Non-Capital Expenditure

Sources of non-capital expenditure
We have seen in earlier chapters how the basis for meeting the cost of the health services changed from local taxation, with a minor fraction of the cost met by central grants, to central taxation supplemented by local taxation. The share met by local taxation decreased, particularly since the health boards became responsible for the services in April 1971 and ultimately, in the period 1973-1976 the contribution from local taxation was phased out entirely. With the local rates no longer meeting any part of the cost, the sources of public finance in Ireland for the health services are now the Exchequer, the Hospitals Sweepstakes and health contributions from eligible persons. A new external source of finance has been introduced under EEC Regulations governing liability for the cost of health care for insured members and pensioners.

The trend since 1973 in the proportions of non-capital expenditure met from the different sources is set out in the Table on page 86.

It will be seen that, at the present time, all but 5·5 per cent of expenditure is met from the Exchequer.

85

Table 1—Sources of Health Funds

Source	Percentage of cost met from each source				
	Year 1973/4	9 months to 31.12.74	Year 1975	Year 1976	Year 1977
	%	%	%	%	%
Exchequer	80·5	86·6	92·4	94·0	94·5
Rates	13·9	8·1	2·3	0·6	Nil
Hospitals sweepstakes	0·6	0·5	0·7	0·6	0·5
Health contributions	3·8	3·7	3·7	4·0	4·0
Recovery of cost under regulations of the EEC	1·2	1·1	0·9	0·8	1·0

Distribution of non-capital health funds to different agencies
The Exchequer funds are voted each year and the amount is shown in the Volume of Estimates. The income from health contributions is shown as an appropriation-in-aid to the Health Vote in that volume. In effect, this means that income becomes available, with the Exchequer contribution, for distribution by the Minister for Health.

The Vote for Health sets out the broad headings for which the funds are to be used, and the classes of agencies to which the funds are distributed. The Volume of Estimates for 1978 allows for a distribution in that year of non-capital funds as shown in Table 2 on page 87.

Health board finances
The health boards are, of course, the major agencies in providing the services (indeed, the grants paid to most of the other agencies by the Department are for services provided by them 'on behalf of health boards'). Therefore, the financial relationships between the Minister and the health boards are the most significant feature in the financial arrangements for the

Table 2—Distribution of 1978 funds by Agencies

Purpose and agencies	Total allocation £m.	Percentage of Estimate %
Expenses of Department of Health	2·5	0·69
Grants to health boards (including balances for previous years)	258·5	71·79
Grants to voluntary hospitals, homes and agencies (including balances for previous years)	97·6	27·10
Developmental, consultative and advisory bodies	0·4	0·10
Grant to Health Education Bureau	1·0	0·28
Miscellaneous	0·1	0·03
Total Estimate	360·1	100·00
less appropriations-in-aid	20·0	
Net Total	340·1	

services. These relationships are governed by part IV of the Health Act, 1970. The Minister prescribes a standard form of accounts for health boards, appoints Local Government auditors to examine the accounts of the boards, submits the Abstracts of Accounts to the Houses of the Oireachtas and may require the boards to submit to him estimates of receipts and expenditure. A health board is not permitted to incur expenditure for any service or purpose beyond the sum fixed for a particular period by the Minister, and the chief executive officer of a board is charged particularly with responsibility for seeing that this restriction is observed.

Distribution of non-capital expenditure by programmes
Health activities are grouped into programmes and sub-

programmes and each of the health agencies funded as shown above is engaged in work on one or more of these programmes. The division of the 1977 expenditure of all the agencies on each of the programmes was as set out in Table 3.

Table 3–1977 Expenditure by Programmes

| Programme (1) | Expenditure | | Percentage of total net expenditure allocated to programme (4) |
	Total £m. (2)	Net of income* £m. (3)	
Community protection	7·60	7·47	2·3
Community health services	46·48	45·28	13·8
Community welfare	27·56	27·10	8·3
Rehabilitation	1·54	1·52	0·5
Psychiatric	46·50	42·35	12·9
Mental handicap	22·84	21·83	6·6
Physical handicap	5·73	5·60	1·7
General hospitals	173·03	155·54	47·3
General support	24·28	21·78	6·6
Total for all programmes	355·56	328·47	100·0

Each of these programmes includes a number of services. Appendix C lists these and also shows the division of the total expenditure in 1977 by services.

Analysis of non-capital expenditure by nature of items
The table on page 89 shows the analysis of the 1977 expenditure by the nature of the items on which it was incurred.

Trends in non-capital health expenditure
Until 31 March 1971 health services were the responsibility of local authorities. The total cost of the health services operated by these authorities, was about £2.7 million in the year to 31 March 1938, and about £5.7 million in the year to 31 March

*In each programme, miscellaneous income accrues from various sources.

Table 4–1977 Expenditure by nature of items.

Item	Gross expenditure on item (£m.)	Percentage of total gross expenditure
1 Pay:		
Nursing and allied	84·1	23·7
Medical and dental	37·5	10·5
Catering, housekeeping and attendants	29·9	8·4
Administrative	16·1	4·5
Paramedical	15·5	4·4
Maintenance	8·0	2·2
Other	5·6	1·6
Superannuation	5·5	1·5
Social welfare contributions (employers)	8·4	2·4
Total Pay	210·6	59·2
2 Non-pay:		
Drugs and medicine	29·5	8·3
Cash allowances	19·1	5·4
Provisions	15·5	4·4
Extern hospitals and homes (subventions and capitation rates) and grants by health boards to voluntary bodies	12·0	3·4
Heat, power and light	9·7	2·7
Finance charges	8·3	2·3
Medical appliances	8·0	2·2
Transport, travelling and subsistence	6·1	1·7
Maintenance (materials and contract work)	5·4	1·5

Laboratory and X-Ray	5·0	1·4
Office equipment and supplies	4·1	1·2
Cleaning and washing materials	3·9	1·1
Other expenses	18·4	5·2
Total non-pay	145·0	40·8
Total expenditure	355·6	100·0
Income	27·1	
Net expenditure	328·9	

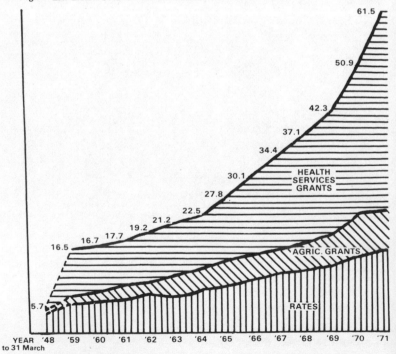

Fig. 5 EXPENDITURE OF HEALTH AUTHORITIES AT CURRENT PRICES (£m)

1948. The reasons for this increase need not be discussed in any detail. It is sufficient to say that the increase was due more to the drop in the value of money than to improvements in the service.

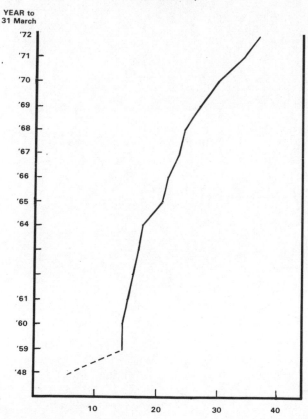

Fig. 6 EXPENDITURE OF HEALTH AUTHORITIES
AT CONSTANT 1953 PRICES
(£ MILLION).

THE HEALTH SERVICES OF IRELAND

Increases in expenditure on local health services since 1948 were at a much greater rate and were caused by two factors, the continuing fall in the value of money and the various extensions of services and improvements in services which were part of national policy. In the last decade of the local authorities' responsibility the increase was particularly marked, as is

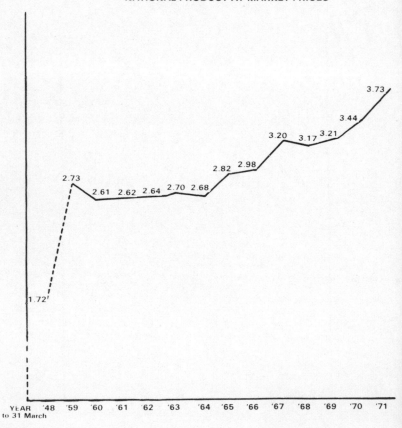

Fig. 7 **EXPENDITURE OF HEALTH AUTHORITIES AS PERCENTAGE OF GROSS NATIONAL PRODUCT AT MARKET PRICES**

illustrated by the graph (page 90). It shows the trend in total expenditure by local health authorities and the proportion in each year met from the rates and from the two Exchequer sources, grants to health authorities and the Agricultural Grant.

To the extent that the expenditure from the Exchequer through the Hospitals Trust Fund to meet deficits of voluntary hospitals is omitted, the graph does not illustrate the full extent of the rise in public expenditure.

If the effect of changing money values is taken out, the increase in expenditure was less spectacular, but still impressive. The graph (page 91) shows the trend at constant 1953 prices, in health expenditure of local authorities from 1948 to 1971.

This rise in expenditure at constant prices was partly met by rising national income but, during the period, the trend in the proportion of the gross national product devoted to the health services was almost continually upward, as is shown by the graph on page 92.

Since the health boards became responsible for the services, the upward trend has continued and in cash terms, has been

Table 5—Trends in Non-capital Health Expenditure since 1971

Year	Expenditure £m.	Expenditure at constant 1971 prices £m.	Percentage of gross national product %
1971/2	86·6	86·6	5·5
1972/3	108·1	99·3	4·7
1973/4	142·8	116·6	5·2
1974[1]	179·6	130·1	6·0
1975	242·6	143·6	6·6
1976	274·6	140·1	6·1
1977 (estimated)	328·0	147·3	6·1

1. Expenditure for the nine-months to the end of 1974 converted to the annual equivalent.

much accentuated. As shown in the table on page 86, the proportion met from direct taxation has increased greatly and the local contribution is now eliminated.

The table on page 93 shows the total expenditure for each year since 1971, in cash terms and at constant prices and the estimated proportion of gross national product (at market prices) spent on health services. These figures are not quite comparable to those in the graphs above because some expenditures not covered by the graphs is included.

Capital Expenditure

Sources of funds
In the past, the main source of monies for capital expenditure was the Hospitals Trust Fund, which has been described on page 15.

In all, the yield for this purpose from the sweepstakes was about £32 million and the fund was used, particularly during

Table 6—Allocation of Capital Expenditure by Categories of hospitals, etc.

Category	Percentage of Total Allocation	
	Period 1933-73	Year 1977
General hospitals	38·8	62·3
Maternity and children's hospitals	7·1	2·0
Infectious disease hospitals	2·4	0·2
Psychiatric hospitals	12·3	11·4
Tuberculosis hospitals	15·3	0·1
Orthopaedic hospitals	2·2	0·6
Mental handicap homes	8·7	9·1
Accommodation for aged	9·9	8·1
Rehabilitation institutions	0·6	0·6
Health clinics	2·7	5·6

the 1930s, to provide many new hospitals and to extend a number of other hospitals. In recent years, however, the income from the sweepstakes has become a much less significant part of the resources for capital expenditure. At present, about 90 per cent of the funds for capital expenditure in the health services is met by central taxation. The total capital allocation for 1977 was £16·5 million and for 1978 it is £20 million.

The total amount of capital expenditure on hospital services from public funds in any year is determined by the allocation given by the Government to the Minister for Health for this purpose. The funds available to him are allocated by the Minister to different agencies and for different purposes. Specific allocations of capital resources are decided on by the Minister for Health. In making his decisions the Minister takes into account the national priorities for different categories of services and the needs of particular areas and particular institutions. In particular, where health board hospitals are concerned in capital development, the views of the health board in relation to priorities are given weight. The Department of Health supervises expenditure of allocated monies. Depending on the scale of expenditure and the type of project, this can vary from involvement in detailed specifications and plans to a general overall specification for accommodation and limits of cost.

The table (p. 94) shows the percentage of the total allocation for the year 1977 for different categories of hospitals and other institutions with, for comparative purposes, the percentage of the total capital expenditure in the period 1933 to 1973 for these purposes.

Health Contributions

Flat-rate contributions
The Health Contributions Act, 1971, introduced a new source of finance to meet part of the cost of the provision of services by health boards. This is a scheme of contributions by persons with limited eligibility (the definition of these is given in Chapter Eight) towards the cost of the services available to them. The scheme of contributions was introduced on 1 October 1971, the rate of contribution then being 15 new

pence per week for insured workers and £7 a year for farmers, for other self-employed persons and for those with private means. At the same time, charges for hospital services formerly payable by those with limited eligibility were abolished. The contributions are collected from insured persons through the Social Welfare stamp, from farmers by the health boards and from others by the Revenue Commissioners.

Although the scheme was essentially designed for those with limited eligibility, some modification had to be provided for because of administrative requirements. As contributions from insured workers were collected as part of the Social Welfare stamp, they fell both on workers with limited eligibility and those with full eligibility. Special categories for whom there was a separate rate of Social Welfare contribution and who were largely in the 'full eligibility' group were entirely exempted from contribitions (these were agricultural labourers and female domestics). However, for those in the general insurance category, it was not practicable to make such exemptions and in this case the health contributions element in the Social Welfare stamp was paid by the employer where the employee had full eligibility. In other cases, of course, the employee met the cost. There were a number of changes in the rates of con-

Table 7—Health contributions—rates and yield

Year	Rate		Yield
	weekly p	yearly £	£m.
1971/2	15	7	1·9
1972/3	15	7	4·7
1973/4	15	7	5·0
1974	15	7	4·2
1975	26	12	8·7
1976	33	15	10·8
1977	39	18	13·3
1978	50	24	16·6 (est.)

tribution since 1971. These are shown in the table (p. 96), which also shows the yield in each year.

The 1971 Act specifically required that all health contributions, in whatever way they are collected, are paid over to the Minister for Health, to be disposed of by him in accordance with Regulations made with the consent of the Minister for Finance. As mentioned earlier, the proceeds of the contributions go to relieve the Health Vote.

Pay-related contributions
This scheme of flat-rate contributions did not represent the scheme of preference and the Act provided for the replacement of this scheme by one under which the contributions would be at a rate relating to income and, in the case of farmers, generally to notional income based on valuation. Such a scheme commenced in April 1979.

The contributions under this new scheme are at the rate of 1 per cent of income, up to a 'ceiling' of £5,500 a year, which will be adjustable with movements in wages. The contributions will be collected with income tax by the Revenue Commissioners, except in the case of most farmers. The health boards will continue to collect the contributions from them.

Under the new scheme, all income earners are liable to pay the health contributions, with the exception of persons with full eligibility and persons in receipt of certain social welfare benefits. Employers continue to be liable to pay health contributions for employees with full eligibility.

Those paying the maximum contribution of £55 a year (i.e. persons with incomes of £5,500 or more a year) are being brought into the scheme with some restriction on eligibility for services. This is described on page 00. The estimated total yield in a full year under the new scheme is £30 million.

The Budgeting System

Now that health costs are met almost entirely from central taxation, budgeting for the health services has increasingly become a part of general national budgeting. What is spent on the health services in any year is governed by the amount allocated to Health in the Government's consideration of the Estimates for the Public Services as a whole. On the basis of Estimates prepared by the Department of Health, a decision is taken by the Government on the allocation for health and this decision determines the level of activity, both non-capital and capital, in the system as a whole and the growth (if any) which is possible in the year.

At this stage, the allocation is on a national basis and its subdivision between the health boards serving the different areas and between different parts of the services is in the control of the Minister for Health and the Department of Health. The Department allocates the funds available between each of the agencies (having kept a small proportion, as shown in Table 2, for its own requirements).

The allocation between different agencies is based on estimates submitted by them and on the general input of information on the services and on needs in different areas. While this input of information is an on-going process throughout the year, the endeavour in recent years has been to concentrate the decisions on the allocations (and accordingly on what developments, if any, are possible in particular areas) into the budgetary cycle. When each health board is notified of its allocation, it is under a statutory obligation to remain within that allocation in its total expenditure, and in its expenditure on particular services (these are set out below). Where grants are paid to other agencies—mainly voluntary hospitals—which provide services on behalf of the health boards, these also are given a fixed allocation and clearly understand that further funds will not be available except to meet circumstances, such as pay awards and increases in prices accepted by the Government, which arise during the year.

The health boards receive some supplementary income from what are described as 'miscellaneous receipts'. The main source of these would be fees from private patients. The voluntary hospitals receive miscellaneous income of a similar kind and also some income from voluntary donations, bequests etc. To the extent that such income is available to the health boards and the voluntary hospitals, they have discretion in devoting it to such of their requirements as they decide. It is not a very high proportion of the total cost so that, in effect, the health agencies are dependent on the funds available from the Department of Health and must work within the approved budgets.

International Comparisons of Health Expenditure

It is difficult to compare the health expenditures of different countries because of problems of definition, but there have been a number of international studies in this field. In 1967, Professor Brian Abel-Smith conducted a study for the World Health Organisation which compared health expenditures in thirteen varied countries. The percentage of gross national product shown in Professor Abel-Smith's study varied from 2·6 in the case of Finland to 4·3 in the case of Israel. The study related only to public expenditure and hence countries with a large private sector in the health field, such as the United States showed a lower percentage of gross national product. Ireland was not a participant in this study but a calculation made by the author showed that we would have been about half-way in the 'league-table' as represented by the proportion of gross national product.

A significant trend was mentioned in Professor Abel-Smith's study and this was that in high-income countries the proportion of gross national product spent on public health services rose, generally at a rate equivalent to 1 per cent or more of gross national product every ten years. This was, indeed, the experience in Ireland during the 1960s.

A table provided by Mr. Robert Maxwell, Administrator to the Special Trustees for St. Thomas's Hospital, London, shows that the international trend has not changed and has indeed become stronger. The trend, and the concern about it, has continued to rise since 1975 and the percentage of gross national product devoted to health care in Sweden and the United States is now at a level of about 10 per cent.

These figures relate to total expenditure, public and private, on health care in the countries concerned. They are not, therefore, comparable to the figures for Ireland shown in Table 5 above. We do not have information on the percentage of gross national product in Ireland spent on private medical care but a rough estimate might be that it would add 1 per cent to each of the figures shown in that table. Perhaps, in relation to the

international trend, the relative stability in recent years shown
in Table 5 in the percentage of gross national product spent on
our public health services might have some significance.

Chapter Eight

Eligibility for Health Services

On the principles of selectivity referred to in the earlier chapters, some people have entitlement to all the health services and the entitlement of others is limited to selected services. Earlier thinking on eligibility was codified in the Health Act, 1970. This defined two groups, those with 'full eligibility' and those with 'limited eligibility', leaving a group of persons with higher incomes who were in neither of these categories. The changes made in April 1979 changed this by simply extending 'limited eligibility' to include the last-mentioned group. However, as will be seen below, some restrictions were made in this extension of eligibility.

Full eligibility
Those with full eligibility are defined as 'adult persons unable without undue hardship to arrange general practitioner, medical and surgical services for themselves and their dependants' and dependants of such persons.[1] It is stated that, where a decision is taken as to whether or not a person comes within this definition 'regard shall be had to the means of the spouse (if any) of that person in addition to the person's own means' (this removed a doubt in the corresponding earlier definition which had permitted the incomes of other working members of the household to be taken into account in taking similar decisions). The criterion, therefore, as to whether a person has or has not full eligibility relates to his ability to pay for family doctor services. Apart from the clarification of those means to be taken into account, this is not much different from the earlier criterion of eligibility for the dispensary service.

The definition of full eligibility is relevant mainly to the general practitioner service which is described in Chapter Ten. The practical operation (and the economics) of this service are

[1]Section 45 of the Health Act, 1970. Adult persons are persons over sixteen years of age (see definition in section 2 of the Health Act, 1947).

dependant on clear specification of those entitled to it. Each health board, therefore, keeps a register of persons with full eligibility which it reviews periodically.

These registers relate simply to entitlement to the general practitioner service, but the definition of 'full eligibility' is used for other services and purposes. In its interpretation for any particular service, there is a clause which permits the chief executive officer of the health board (or one of his subordinates) to exercise discretion and accept a hardship case as entitled.

For some years, the chief executive officers of the eight health boards have agreed on generally applicable guidelines for the decisions on full eligibility. These are reviewed at intervals, usually yearly. The guidelines in operation from 1 January 1979 are set out in Appendix D. This also shows the numbers with full eligibility by county on 31 March 1978 and the general classification of those covered.

The decisions on which individuals have full eligibility are taken by officers of the health board (the board, as a body of members, are prohibited from intervening). The primary decisions are taken locally by a subordinate officer and there is an appeal against refusal.

The Minister for Health has power to make regulations specifying 'a class or classes of persons who shall be deemed to be within the categories' having full eligibility. Such regulations have not been made.

Limited eligibility

The concept of 'limited eligibility' was introduced under Section 46 of the Health Act, 1970. Broadly those included within the concept were persons insured under the Social Welfare Acts (with an income limit for non-manual workers), other persons with yearly means under a fixed limit and farmers with valuations of £60 or less, and dependents of persons in each of these groups. The income limit fixed by the 1970 Act had been revised and stood at £3,000 a year in April 1979. There were complex requirements about social welfare contributions for non-manual workers.

The Health Services (Limited Eligibility) Regulations, 1979 replaced the complex definition in Section 46 of the 1970 Act with a simple statement: 'A person who is without full eligibility shall have limited eligibility for services under this Part (of the 1970 Act)'. Thus the entire population became divided into the group with full eligibility, as it then existed, and the remainder. However, the Health Services Regulations, 1979 placed some restrictions on the 'limited eligibility' services available to the category with incomes at or above the level of £5,500 a year (this limit relates to incomes in the tax year ended on 5 April 1979 and, as indicated above, will be reviewed each year).

General provisions on eligibility
Health boards have power to require persons to make declarations in relation to means and to verify such declarations. Where a person is recorded as entitled to a particular service, he is required to notify the board of any change in his circumstances which disentitles him to the service and if he obtains the service and it is found out that he was not entitled, he may be charged for it. There are penalties also for false statements, etc., in relation to eligibility.[2]

The services: eligibility
Eligibility for most of the major branches of the health services is formally expressed by reference to full eligibility and limited eligibility but, because of the sub-division now of the latter concept, it is more convenient to discuss eligibility by reference to the following three categories.
Category 1: This category covers persons with full eligibility, as described above. Those in it are entitled to the full range of health services without charge, including general practitioner services. Medical cards are issued to persons in this category for presentation when services are needed. Somewhat less than 40 per cent of the population are in this category.
Category 2: This covers persons, other than those in Category 1, whose income in the year ended 5 April 1979 was less than £5,500. Persons in this category are entitled without charge to hospital services (both maintenance and treatment) in public wards, to special services in out-patient clinics and maternity and infant welfare services. A person in this category is also

[2]Sections 48 to 50 and 75 of Health Act, 1970.

entitled to a subsidy towards the cost of maintenance in an approved private hospital or home where he chooses this instead of a public hospital. Those in this category are also entitled to a refund of part of the cost of prescribed drugs and medicines (see page 124). About 45 per cent of the population is in this category.

Category 3: The remainder of the population, that is persons whose income in the year ended 5 April 1979 was £5,500 or more, are in this category. They are entitled without charge to hospital services on the same basis as those in Category 2 except that they are liable to pay hospital consultants' fees. They are also entitled to avail themselves of the scheme of subsidies towards the cost of maintenance in approved private hospitals or homes and to the refund scheme for drugs and medicines.

As regards Categories 2 and 3, where a husband and wife have separate incomes, the eligibility of each is assessed separately. Where a dependent spouse has no income, he or she will be in the same category as the income-earner. The rule applicable to children under sixteen years of age is that, if both parents are in Category 2, so are the children but if either parent is in Category 3, then the children are regarded as being in that category.

To distinguish between those in Categories 2 and 3 for the purpose of hospital services, special arrangements are made by health boards. The object of this is to identify those in the former category on the basis of evidence of income in the preceding tax year. It involves the issue of hospital services cards to those in Category 2 or, where this has not been done before admission to hospital, the identification of the category at the time of admission.

There are a number of services for which this categorising of the population is irrelevant. For example, treatment of infectious diseases is available free to all. Hospital treatment, both in-patient and out-patient is also available without charge for all children under sixteen years of age suffering from certain long-term ailments. Neither is there any means test for health examinations for pupils of national schools and health examinations at child health clinics or for out-patients specialist services for defects noticed at such examinations.

Table 1—Pattern of eligibility[1]

Service or Item	Category		
	1	2	3
General practitioner care ..	F	—	—
Drugs and medicines			
long term ailments ..	F	F	F
other	F	P	P
District nursing	F	C	C
Home helps	C	C	C
Infectious diseases			
immunisation	F	F	F
treatment (hospital) ..	F	F	F
maintenance allowances ..	F	C	C
Maternity and infant care			
medical and midwifery	F	F	—
maternity grants ..	F	—	—
milk for mothers and			
children	F	—	—
Child health examinations			
pre-school	F	F	F
for national school pupils	F	F	F
Dental, ophthalmic and aural			
children	F	C	C
adults	F	—	—
Hospital care (in-patient and out-patient)			
long-term defects			
in children	F	F	F
other	F	F	P
Welfare homes	F	—	—
Rehabilitation	F	F	F
Allowances to disabled			
persons	F	—	—
Screening tests	F	F	F

[1]F denotes full entitlement, P partial entitlement and C entitlement subject to conditions.

The table (p. 105) shows for those in each of the three categories the general pattern of entitlement to services. The letter 'F' denotes full entitlement to the service without charge, the letter 'P' denotes partial entitlement (by way of subvention or limited in some other way) and the letter 'C' denotes entitlement subject to conditions. This table does not of course demonstrate all the nuances and conditions for eligibility. It merely shows the pattern. The chapters on individual services give more detail, but individual issues of eligibility can be determined only by the officers of the health boards. The table relates to eligibility in the context of the services provided by the health boards. It does not relate to the services offered by the Voluntary Health Insurance Board. When account is taken of these, the pattern of services in this country can fairly be described as offering to all the capability of avoiding oppressive direct expenditure on health care.

Chapter Nine

Voluntary Health Insurance

Voluntary health insurance as a means of providing for wide classes of the population had been the subject of considerable discussion before the extended local authority services under the Health Act of 1953 were decided upon. The new hospital and specialist services under that Act were designed to cater for the needs of some 85 per cent of the population. When these services had been introduced, there remained the issue as to whether or not anything should be done to sponsor or encourage voluntary health insurance, particularly for those outside the 'Health Act' classes. To further the resolution of this issue, the Minister for Health appointed a special advisory body in January 1955.

Report of advisory body
In their report to the Minister in May 1956,[1] this advisory body found that voluntary health insurance benefits were provided only on a very limited scale in this country. The following is an extract from the relevant paragraph of the report:

'7 . . . . Few of the commercial insurance companies transact health insurance business and none does so to any material extent. One company introduced a scheme in 1953 offering hospital, medical and surgical benefits. It subsequently increased by 50 per cent the premium rates initially charged but, notwithstanding this, decided to terminate the scheme after about two years' experience. Some sickness benefits are provided through Friendly Societies of which about 100 are registered: of these some 30, with a total membership of approximately 17,000, disburse sickness benefits in one form or another, and the total amount paid each year is about £17,000. In addition, there are a number of schemes associated with particular firms or organisations which

---

[1]Report of Advisory Body on Voluntary Health Insurance Scheme (Prl. 3571). Published by the Stationery Office, Dublin.

provide sickness benefits for their members, generally in the form of contributions towards hospital and medical expenses.'

In approaching their terms of reference, the advisory body assumed that the primary objective on which they were asked to advise was protection against the high and unforeseeable cost of ill-health and not against the minor costs which can readily be allowed for in the family budget. The benefits which the advisory body thought should be given under such a scheme were maintenance in hospital or nursing home, surgical and medical fees (in accordance with a graduated scale for major, intermediate and minor operations), maternity benefit, drugs and medicines for hospital in-patients, medical and surgical appliances, and various specialist services for in-patients in hospital. The body recommended that specialist medical services given outside hospitals and dental treatment be not covered. They also thought that no benefit should be included for the supply of drugs and medicines, except for persons in hospital. The report recommended that in any scheme there should be a waiting period of three months except for claims arising from accidents and that the insurance should be on the basis of annual contracts.

Having considered the possibilities of the operation of their scheme by various types of agencies and having commented on the practice in other countries, the body advised:

'We are not aware that there are any interests in this country prepared to establish a health insurance scheme of the kind mentioned in our terms of reference and if a scheme is to be introduced, the State must take the initiative. A scheme could be administered by a Department of State, but we think it would have a wider appeal to the public if it were administered by a company such as we describe.'

The company envisaged by the advisory body was one which would be guaranteed by the State, at the commencement at least, and which would not be obliged to comply with the provisions in the Insurance Acts relating to the licensing of insurance companies.

On the basis of the figures available to it, the body reached the general conclusion that, although a voluntary health insurance scheme would increase the income of voluntary hospitals, the increase was unlikely to be appreciable in relation either to the total income of those hospitals or to their annual deficits.

A calculation in the Report of the Advisory Body shows that at the time it was prepared, there were some 457,000 persons not entitled to the health services under the Health Act of 1953 and thus potential clients for a voluntary health insurance scheme. The body thought that if persons eligible for Health Act services who might be disposed to become members were included, the total potential number of participants would be in the region of 500,000. They cautioned, however, that 'one would have to assume that the number of persons who would be likely to join a scheme, particularly at its commencement, would be considerably less than the figure mentioned.'

The recommendations of the advisory body were accepted with some exceptions and were the basis of the Voluntary Health Insurance Act, 1957.

The Voluntary Health Insurance Board
Under this Act a new board, the Voluntary Health Insurance Board, was set up. The chairman and other members are appointed by the Minister and have a five-year term of office. There are five members.[2] The board is charged with providing health insurance schemes, including a minimum scheme prescribed by the Minister. It is a non-profit-making body, any surplus on its income being devoted to the reduction of premiums or increases in benefits.[3] To cover its preliminary expenses, an interest-bearing loan of £25,000 from the Minister for Health was provided for (only £13,200 of this was, in fact, called upon).

The board's schemes
When the board commenced business in October, 1957, it offered three separate schemes. The basic scheme provided for

[2]The full provisions on the constitution, etc., of the board are in sections 3 to 21 of the Act.
[3]Section 4 (4) of the Act.

maintenance benefit at the rate of £6 6s. 0d. a week, with further benefits to cover medical and surgical fees and other expenses in hospitals. Two other schemes were introduced at the same time, giving higher benefits of the same type for higher premiums. There was no provision in any of these schemes for coverage for normal maternity care.

After some years' operation of the schemes of this type, the board changed over to more flexible provisions, whereby the policy-holder could choose the cover which he wished to take out for maintenance or treatment. However, its new schemes, as introduced in April 1979, revert to the concept of three general plans. These are designed to complement the changes in eligibility for public services described in Chapter Eight.

The Board's Plan A is intended to cover the full charge (after allowing for the public subsidy) for private or semi-private accommodation in public hospitals; Plan B covers this and also care up to semi-private level in private hospitals and nursing homes; and Plan C is designed for those who wish to have a choice of private accommodation in any hospital in the state.

The new plans offer better provision for out-patient care, day surgery, special nursing and ambulance charges and, for the first time, cover hospital costs for normal maternity care.

The premiums for the board's schemes are graded in relation to the cover given and the number of dependants of the insured person. Full particulars of the schemes and the rules and conditions governing them are given in a brochure issued free by the board.

Numbers insured

The numbers covered by the board's scheme have steadily increased since it commenced business. On 28 February 1958, the membership was 23,238; on 28 February 1961, it was 105,526; in 1964, it was 195,189; in 1967, it was 288,496; in 1971, it was 436,144 and on 28 February 1978 the total covered had reached 645,165.

In the financial year 1976-77, the board paid out a total of £10,983,965 in claims; its administrative expenses amounted to £868,563 which represented 7·2 per cent of the total income. The board, in its annual reports, publishes very interesting analyses of its claims experience, showing the major diseases for which claims are made and categorising the claimants by age group and otherwise.

Occupation of subscribers
The table below, taken from the board's report for the year to 28 February 1977 shows the occupations of the subscribers at that date (these, with their dependants, make up the total membership referred to earlier).

Table 1—Occupations of VHI subscribers

Occupation	Numbers
Commercial and industrial	82,310
Professional	27,983
Teachers	18,270
Civil Service	13,312
Agriculture	13,865
Banks	8,567
Religious	9,769
Local Authorities	1,545
Insurance	2,302
Garda Síochána	4,695
Defence Forces	810
Miscellaneous	28,622
Total	212,050

Licensing of other insurers [4]
By the Voluntary Health Insurance Act, health insurance was freed from the controls exercised on insurance businesses generally under the Insurance Acts 1909 to 1953. Instead, it was made necessary for any person (with some exceptions—the most important being trade unions and friendly societies) wishing to provide health insurance to hold a licence from the Minister for Health. These licences are issued only for limited types of insurance schemes which would not be seriously competitive with those of the Voluntary Health Insurance Board.

[4]Sections 22 to 25 of the Act.

To provide health insurance without a licence (where such is required) or to pay a subscription or premium to a person doing this is an offence.

Income tax relief on voluntary health premiums
Money paid as subscriptions or premiums for voluntary health insurance may be claimed for deduction from income in the calculation of income tax.[5] The full amount paid is deductible so that, at current rates of taxation, those liable for income tax at the standard rate obtain relief to the extent of about one-third of what they pay for voluntary health insurance.

Income tax refunds for health expenses
Income tax payers may obtain some relief on heavy private expenditure on health care through a scheme operated by the Revenue Commissioners.[6] If, in any year, the amount of expenditure for an individual which is not met from public funds or insurance is greater than £50, any excess qualifies for a special rebate of income tax. These limits apply to each dependant of the taxpayer individually and not to the total costs incurred by the taxpayer on himself and his dependants. A separate calculation is made for each. The scheme extends to most forms of medical and ancillary treatment but not to routine ophthalmic or dental treatment.

Claims under the scheme are made after the end of the tax year in question and the refund is calculated at the standard taxation rate. For example, if there has been expenditure of £160 on a taxpayer or his dependant, he will get a refund of £38·50 (£160 less £50=£110 @ 35p in the £ £38·50). The rebate only applies, of course, if that amount of tax, or more, has been paid. The scheme is thus a useful aid to those who pay income tax.

International Federation of Voluntary Health Service Funds
This international body has its headquarters in Ireland and is incorporated here under the International Health Bodies (Corporate Status) Act, 1971. The aims and purposes of the

---

[5] Section 4 of Finance Act, 1955.
[6] Under section 12 of the Finance Act, 1967, as amended by section 7 of the Finance Act, 1969.

Federation, which had its origins in a decision taken at the first International Conference on Voluntary Health Insurance held in Dublin in 1966, are to assist individuals in obtaining health services and for this purpose to promote the development and study of voluntary non-profit health services throughout the world.

Membership of the Federation, which is a non-profit-making body, is open to organisations carrying out, or co-ordinating, voluntary health services on a non-profit basis, other organisations interested in voluntary non-profit health services, and persons interested in voluntary non-profit health services. The Voluntary Health Insurance Board is a member of the Federation. In all, about 90 organisations in various countries are members.

Chapter Ten
Health Care in the Community

This chapter deals with those health services in which care is provided outside hospitals and other institutions and with related welfare services. A series of programmes is designed so as to enable the community to enjoy a high level of personal health in a healthy environment. These are

—the community protection programme (covering the prevention of infectious diseases, child health examinations, food hygiene and food standards, drug controls, health education and other preventive services);

—the community health services programme (covering general practitioner services, including the supply of drugs and medicines and schemes for subsidising drug purchases, home nursing services, domiciliary maternity services and dental, ophthalmic and aural services);

—the community welfare programme (including cash payments to disabled persons and to persons with certain infectious diseases, home help and meals-on-wheels services, grants to voluntary welfare agencies, supply of free milk, maintenance of deprived children and welfare homes for the aged).

The Community Protection Programme

Earlier chapters have described how preventive health services were developed in conjunction with environmental protection by the local sanitary authorities, working first under the Local Government Board and later under the Department of Local Government and Public Health. Responsibility for these groups of services at central level was split in 1947, when the Department of Health became responsible for the services relating to personal health and the Department of Local Government retained broad responsibility for services related to the environment. The division was made roughly between those services in which the medical content was predominant and those where engineering was the major factor. This split of responsibility is now reflected at local level, where the health boards have taken

114

over from the local authorities the responsibility for the personal health services, but the environmental services have been left with the latter authorities. The medical officers of the health boards still, however, advise the local authorities on medical aspects of housing, planning and development, water supplies, sewage disposal and other environmental problems. The main direct responsibilities of the health boards in the field of preventive health relate to infectious disease control, food hygiene and food standards, the quality and safety of drugs, the arranging of 'screening tests' and general health education.

Infectious disease control
Communicable diseases no longer present the same problems as they did for many decades. Fortunately, the incidence and the mortality rates from most of these diseases have declined so as to become negligible. The control of infectious diseases, for which the public health services were first organised, thus tends to pass into the background behind the new responsibilities of the health boards. This may be attributed to a number of factors, of which the more important were the development of vaccines and other prophylactic agents, improved sanitation and hygiene, new and improved drugs and the generally greater awareness within the community of the value of these preventive measures.

The infectious disease service, however, remains an important part of the community care programme and its continued smooth operation is essential if a re-emergence of major problems arising from infectious diseases is to be avoided. The elements on which the effectiveness of the service depends are notification, diagnosis and treatment (available without means test), prevention of the spread of infection, immunisation and vaccination, and the payment of maintenance allowances. There is a considerable body of law on these matters, mainly based on Part IV of the Health Act, 1947 and the regulations made under that Part. The provisions of this body of law are summarised in Appendix E.

New problems were presented for the infectious disease service with the increase in international travel. This trend, and in particular the rise in the numbers holidaying abroad each year, has called for greater organisation and greater alertness in precautions to safeguard the health of travellers and those with whom they come into contact. Responsibilities in this field rest mainly on those health boards whose areas include the major airports and seaports, but as most modern journeys, even from far-off countries, can be completed within the incubation periods of the most dangerous infectious diseases, all health boards must be watchful. Information leaflets are available to travellers, medical practitioners and travel agencies outlining the possible dangers to health in visiting other countries, particularly those with warm climates, and the precautions which should be taken by travellers.

Prophylactic campaigns have concentrated on smallpox vaccination, diphtheria immunisation, BCG vaccination against tuberculosis, poliomyelitis vaccination and, more recently, vaccination against rubella (German measles).

Tuberculosis
In the first half of this century, tuberculosis was probably the most feared disease in Ireland. The incidence was severe and the death rate high. The disease attacked mainly the young and active and its tragic effects were often accentuated by its spread within families. Happily, this picture has now changed. The number of newly-discovered cases of tuberculosis is falling each year and eradication of the disease from the community now seems an attainable goal. The death rate from the disease, which was 145 per 100,000 of the population in 1927 and 124

Table 1 – Trend of tuberculosis cases and deaths

Year	Respiratory cases	Non-respiratory cases	Total cases	Deaths
1961	2,395	615	3,010	420
1966	1,537	391	1,928	339
1971	943	295	1,238	183
1976	886	175	1,061	158

in 1947, had fallen to 24 in 1957 and to 5 in 1976. This fall in the death rate was accompanied by a fall in the number of cases and there was a marked shift in the incidence of disease to the older age groups, particularly in the case of men. The trend in new cases and deaths since 1961 is shown in the table (p. 116).

In the organisation of the services, tuberculosis is the most significant of the infectious diseases and the responsibility for organising local schemes for the detection of cases of this disease remains an important, if diminishing, part of the work of the medical officers. It is their duty to try to identify the sources of infection, to see that contacts are examined and to arrange for treatment. This side of the work in relation to tuberculosis is centred on clinics and includes a considerable amount of field work. The legal powers required for this work are incorporated in the law for infectious diseases generally which is referred to above.

BCG vaccination against tuberculosis was introduced in 1949, when the National BCG Committee, a voluntary body formed at the request of the Minister for Health, commenced operations. The operation of vaccination schemes is now mainly a matter for the health boards.

Supervision of food and drugs
As part of their duties in controlling the spread of infectious diseases, health authorities have for long had functions in supervising the hygiene of food supplies. For the general well-being of the public, they have also had functions in relation to the quality and safety of food and drugs. Because our modern way of living is so dependent on processed and prepared foods and on an increasing variety of drugs and medicines, the efficacy of these controls is becoming increasingly important. Health boards now have a varied battery of legal powers in operating the controls in these fields.

Hygiene in the manufacture, preparation, sale and serving of food is governed by the Food Hygiene Regulations, 1950 to 1971. The Regulations, which, with the other legal provisions referred to in these paragraphs, are summarised in Appendix F, include a general prohibition of the sale of unfit food and give authority for the seizure of unfit food and power to stop the importation of such food. They also provide for the registration of food premises. The enforcement of the Regulations is mainly in the hands of the health boards, acting through their medical officers and their health inspectors, who have special skills in this field.[1]

The basic provisions on the general quality of food and drugs sold to the public are contained in the Sale of Food and Drugs Acts, 1875 to 1936. These were designed to prevent the sale of food or drugs which were injurious to health or 'not of the nature, substance or quality demanded by the purchaser.' Under these and later Acts, there is also provision for fixing chemical standards for foods and power to make regulations controlling the use of preservatives and colouring matters. The enforcement of these provisions also is mainly in the hands of the health inspectors.

The sale and distribution of poisons and dangerous drugs are subject to a number of statutory controls. The earliest of these dates back to 1851, when controls were introduced specifically on the sale of arsenic. The object of the legislation on poisons is to channel their sale through properly controlled outlets (mainly pharmaceutical chemists' shops) and to ensure that proper records are kept. There are specific provisions in relation to dangerous narcotic drugs, and, more recently, a number of regulations have been brought in to restrict the sale of several drugs and medicines so that they may not be issued except on prescription.

The National Drugs Advisory Board was established[2] in July 1966 to provide a service to monitor newly-introduced medicinal products to check their safety for human use. The Board is also responsible for collecting and disseminating information on side-effects and reactions associated with drugs already in use, and for furnishing advice on precautions and restrictions in the marketing and use of such drugs. The Board has twelve members, appointed by the Minister. The service provided by the Board in relation to the assessment of drugs for safety was for a number of years a voluntary one, operated with the co-operation of the pharmaceutical industry. The in-

[1] Health inspectors are appointed after a four-year training course, which is organised by the Health Inspectors Training Board, a body established by the Minister and financed by the health boards.

[2] Under the National Drugs Advisory Board (Establishment) Order, 1966, made under the Health (Corporate Bodies) Act, 1961.

troduction of a product authorisation scheme under the European Communities (Proprietary Medicinal Products) Regulations, 1974 and a scheme for the licensing of manufacturing and wholesale activities have placed these arrangements on a statutory basis.

Information on adverse reactions to drugs is obtained from practising doctors, from health administrations in other countries, and from the World Health Organisation.

Drug abuse has become an increasing problem in Ireland. In May 1971, a working party established by the Minister for Health reported on this[3] and made a number of recommendations to combat the problem, including the improvement of statutory controls and the maintenance of full liaison by the health authorities with the police and others with responsibilities in the matter. The importance of education and publicity in relation to the problem was stressed, as was the need for a comprehensive programme for the rehabilitation of abusers of drugs. Most of the recommendations of the working party have been acted on and the Misuse of Drugs Act, 1977, which provides a comprehensive legal backing for the control of drug abuse, reflects their recommendations. This Act replaced the Dangerous Drugs Act, 1934.

Child health examinations

Over a period of about fifty years, the local health authorities had developed a school health examination scheme for pupils of national schools and a child welfare clinic service (for children up to the age of six). These services were examined by a study group appointed by the Minister for Health, whose report was published in 1968.[4] The study group recommended that the existing services become a co-ordinated child health service and made several detailed recommendations on its organisation and scope. Perhaps the most important of these were:

scheduled medical examinations should be available to each child at the age of 6 months, 1 year and 2 years;

in urban areas with a population of 5,000 or more, these scheduled medical examinations should be carried out in

[3] Report of Working Party on Drug Abuse, published by the Stationery Office.
[4] *The Child Health Services*, (Stationery Office).

clinics by doctors on the medical officer's staff and, in some smaller towns, similar arrangements could operate;

the school should continue to be used as the basic centre for school health examinations, which would continue to be carried out by local medical officers;

in rural areas and in towns without clinics, the scheduled medical examinations for pre-school children should be undertaken by general practitioners under agreements with the health authorities;

the former aim of three routine medical examinations during a child's national school career should be replaced by a system under which there would be a comprehensive medical inspection of all children between the sixth and seventh birthdays, routine annual screening by the district nurse for vision, posture and cleanliness, audiometric testing of special groups, selected medical examinations of nine-year-old children and the examination in any year of a child referred by the parent, teacher or district nurse, or a child due for re-examination.

The Health Act, 1970, made changes in the law necessary to give effect to recommendations of the working party[5] and the Minister for Health in that year announced that he had accepted the main recommendations. A circular to the local health authorities in July 1970, set out a programme within the period 1970 to 1974 to implement them. The programme provided initially for the development of the pre-school examination service in the towns with a population of 5,000 and over and the restructuring of the school health examination service as recommended. The responsibility for giving effect to this programme is now, of course, one for the health boards.

While there is power in the Health Act, 1970,[6] to bring into the scope of the school health examination service a school which is not a national school on the request of its governing body, such an extension of the service is not an immediate prospect.

[5] Section 66.
[6] Section 66(3).

Health education

The above measures relate to the actions of the public authorities in protecting the community against specific problems. However, over a much wider field, there is a responsibility on those authorities to aid and guide those in the community in protecting health and avoiding illness. Much of this is, of course, done through the direct contacts between the medical officers, nurses and other staff of the health boards with the people; much is also done through use of the mass media of communications.

Because television, radio and the major newspapers are organised on a national basis, the major health publicity campaigns on these media were originally arranged direct by the Department. New developments in the services were publicised and material issued from time to time on specific problems. The Department also published a wide variety of leaflets.

As well as providing information and advice in relation to particular diseases and health problems, the Minister and the health boards have the responsibility to let the public have information on the health services available and on the rules governing eligibility for them. A general summary of the services is available from the Department of Health and more detailed information on them is contained in the Guide to the Social Services.[7] Health boards have the responsibility to make information available on the local arrangements for the services.

The development of arrangements for health education is probably the greatest priority in the health system. Recognition of this led in January 1975 to the establishment of the Health Education Bureau. This is a corporate body with responsibility for organising health education programmes and for acting as the co-ordinating agency for the many voluntary bodies acting in this field. The Bureau has a board of ten members, appointed by the Minister for Health, and employs its own staff to organise health education programmes. The importance of this body's work is reflected in the increase of the budget allocated to it from £300,000 in 1976 to £400,000 in 1977 and to £1m for 1978.

[7]Published by the Stationery Office.

The Community Health Services Programme

General practitioner care

The responsibility of the health boards in organising care at general practitioner level extends only to those with full eligibility, now representing just under 40 per cent of the population.

The arrangements for providing general medical care were radically re-organised in 1972. The salaried dispensary service described earlier was replaced by a new service based on the principle that, where practicable, the eligible person will be offered a choice of doctor.[8]

The new scheme in nearly all areas is based on agreements with participating doctors[9] (rather than on the employment of doctors as officers, as in the case of the dispensary service). The form of agreement is a standard one. It sets out the obligations of the participating practitioner on the one hand and of the health board on the other. Only those practitioners entitled to participate in the scheme, or accepted for participation in it, can enter into agreements and choice by eligible persons is limited to those doctors who have agreements. On the commencement of the new service, doctors in practice had an automatic right of entry. Other general practitioners do not have automatic right of entry. Some may acquire such a right but, in general, new practitioners are admitted only where there is an accepted vacancy and admission is on the basis of open competition. Group practice is allowed within the scheme and is, indeed, encouraged by certain features of it.

Payment under the agreements is on the basis of fees for services, with the rates varying for surgery fees and for various kinds of domiciliary visits (there are higher rates for out-of-hours calls and for distant calls). It is part of the normal contract that the medical practitioner will provide adequate surgery and waiting room facilities and that, in these arrangements, he will not discriminate between public and private patients. However, it is also envisaged that the use of premises such as clinics and dispensaries owned by the health board can be arranged. For islands and a few remote areas where choice

[8]See section 58 of the Health Act, 1970.
[9]These are made under section 26 of the Health Act, 1970.

of doctor is impracticable, the service, like the dispensary service, is arranged through the employment of officers by the health boards.

A full description of these arrangements is given in Appendix G.

Supply of drugs, medicines and appliances
Under the dispensary service, most of the doctors did their own dispensing from stocks of drugs which were kept at the dispensary and replenished by making official requisitions. Where the doctor did not himself dispense, the drugs were issued by a pharmacist at the dispensary. This arrangement too was fundamentally changed in 1972. Now the retail pharmaceutical chemists are the main channels of supply for drugs, medicines and appliances prescribed for eligible persons. Normally, a doctor participating in the new service issues a prescription on a special form and this can be fulfilled by any pharmacist who has an agreement under the service. The pharmacist is recouped the cost to him of the drugs and is paid a fee for dispensing them.

Where the operation of this system of supply would cause hardship, either because there is no retail pharmaceutical chemist in an area or because of special circumstances in the case of a particular patient, it is part of the doctor's contract that he will arrange for the supply of drugs, etc. He is paid a special annual fee for this responsibility. He requisitions his drugs from a convenient retail pharmacist working in the scheme.

These new arrangements for the supply of drugs and medicines are also described fully in Appendix G.

General Medical Services (Payments) Board[10]
The calculation of payments for the services of doctors and pharmacists under the service, the making of such payments, the verification of the accuracy and reasonableness of claims and the compilation of statistics and information on the services, are carried out for the health boards by a joint board, the General Medical Services (Payments) Board. Most of the

[10]Established under the General Medical Services (Payments) Board (Establishment) Order, 1972.

members of this Board are officers of health boards, the others being from the Department of Health.

The claims from doctors and pharmacists under the service are processed through a computer and, on the basis of the information provided, the scheme is monitored regularly by the Board. Each year a comprehensive report is published giving information and statistics on the operation of the scheme. The report for the year 1977 shows that at the end of that year 1,302 doctors and 1,106 pharmacies were registered, the number of persons in the scheme then was 1,233,150, the amount paid in fees to participating doctors in 1977 was almost £11m., the amount paid for medicines was £22·2m., the overall payment per patient was £27.59, and almost 80 per cent of the persons covered by the scheme received services in the year.

Drugs, medicines and appliances for persons with limited eligibility

The 'drug refund scheme' operated by the health boards is designed to insulate those with limited eligibility against having to meet from their own resources heavy expenditure on prescribed drugs, medicines and appliances. Expenditure over a fixed limit any month will be refunded by the health board. At present the arrangement is that expenditure over £5 but less than £8 in a month is met to the extent of 50 per cent and expenditure over £8 is met in full. This refund scheme relates to drugs purchased through the ordinary channels and is based on receipts obtained from the retail pharmacists. From April 1979 this scheme applies to the entire population except for those using the general medical service described above.

Drugs, etc. for long-term ailments

For persons suffering from diseases or disabilities of a permanent or long-term nature listed in regulations made by the Minister for Health, there are arrangements for the free supply of drugs.[11] This scheme is available to all income groups. The list of diseases and disabilities to which it applies at present are mental handicap, mental illness (in children under sixteen), phenylketonuria, cystic fibrosis, spina bifida, hydrocephalus,

[11]Section 59(3) of the Health Act, 1970.

haemophilia, cerebral palsy, diabetes mellitus, diabetes in-
sipidus, epilepsy, multiple sclerosis, muscular dystrophies,
parkinsonism and acute leukaemia in children. This scheme
also operates through the retail pharmaceutical chemists, who
supply the drugs prescribed and make claims for the cost of the
drugs and their charges on the health boards.

Home nursing
Nursing at community level was first developed by voluntary
organisations, particularly the Queen's Institute of District
Nursing in Ireland. Later, there developed, side by side with the
nurses of the voluntary agencies, a corps of public health
nurses attached to the offices of the county medical officers,
with duties mainly in the public health service. The Health Act,
1947, gave health authorities power to appoint nurses for district duties and, in the nineteen-fifties, the authorities commenced the development of this service. Additional impetus was
given by a circular issued by the Department in June 1966,
which defined the objectives of this service and specified the
aims in developing it. The general objective of the service was
stated as being to make public health nursing available to individuals and to families in each area throughout the country.
More specifically, the objective was defined in the following
terms:

'The object should be to provide such domiciliary midwifery
services as may be necessary, general domiciliary nursing,
particularly for the aged, and, at least equally important, to
attend to the public health care of children, from infancy to
the end of the school-going period. The nurses should
provide health education in the home and assist local
medical practitioners in the care of patients who need nursing care but who do not require treatment in an institution—whether for medical or social reasons. The aim
should be to integrate the district nursing service with the
general practitioner, hospital in-patient and out-patient services, so that the nurse will be able to fulfil the important
function of an essential member of the community health
team, and carry out her duties in association with hospital
staffs and other doctors in her district.'

The home nursing service is available generally only to persons with full eligibility but can also be made available to 'such other categories of persons and for such purposes as may be specified by the Minister'.[12]

In 1977 there were 1,045 public health nurses (877 on district duties) which represents one for each 3,050 of population. The aim is to have one nurse for each 2,600 of population.

Maternity and infant care services

The health boards provide a service for medical attendance at general practitioner level on maternity cases and on infants up to the age of six weeks, in the case of those with full eligibility or those in category 2 (as described in Chapter Eight).[13] The service is provided through private medical practitioners under agreements with the health boards. This service also is based on the principle of choice of doctor. There is a standard form of agreement worked out by the Department. The medical practitioner undertakes to attend on any woman accepted by him. He attends during the ante-natal period, at the birth if he thinks it necessary (or if his services are called for by the midwife) and for the period of six weeks after the confinement. The services given normally include at least four visits before the confinement and two after it. Usually the same doctor will attend the infant, carrying out at least one medical examination during the first six weeks of life. The health board pays the fees for attendance on cases under the agreement.

In Dublin, an arrangement is made under which the staffs of the three maternity hospitals provide the same kind of services as are provided under the agreements with general practioners. The hospitals are, in such cases, viewed in the same way as individual participating private practitioners but when accepting services under such an arrangement the woman is not entitled to insist upon having the services of any particular doctor on the hospital staff.

The number of cases attended under this service throughout the country in 1976 was 32,104, representing 47 per cent of all births. However, less than 1 per cent of births took place at home.

---

[12]Section 60 of Health Act, 1970.
[13]Under sections 62 and 63 of Health Act 1970, and article 9 of Health Services Regulations, 1971.

Midwifery services are organised for the same groups in a manner similar to the maternity medical services. Each health board has agreements with midwives. However, with very few domiciliary confinements, this service is now of little significance.

Dental services

The obligation of health boards to provide dental services (and ophthalmic and aural services too) will eventually extend to all those with full eligibility or with limited eligibility.[14] However, the present services arranged by the health boards are concentrated on children (for defects noticed at child health examinations) and those with full eligibility. It has been the policy to restrict the services to these groups until, by adding to the personnel and generally improving the facilities, an adequate service is available for them. In the meantime, for persons insured under the Social Welfare Acts, dental (and optical and aural) benefits are available under a separate scheme administered by the Department of Social Welfare.

The dental services of the health boards are provided mainly through whole-time dentists in their employment. The number of these has increased from 141 in 1971 to 194 in 1978. In some areas, the services provided by this staff are supplemented by the part-time employment of private dental practitioners, who are usually paid on a sessional basis.

The work of the dental service must be largely involved in combating the effects of existing dental decay but it is regarded as important that there should be as much concentration as possible on prevention. The instruction of children in good habits of dental care and oral hygiene is, therefore, a major aim of the service. Dental health campaigns which are conducted by the Dental Health Education Committee of the Irish Dental Association complement the activities of health boards in this field.

Fluoridation

Fluoridation of public water supplies is the most important measure for preventing dental decay. Under the Health (Fluoridation of Water Supplies) Act, 1960, an obligation is

[14]Section 67 of Health Act, 1970.

placed on health boards to arrange for the fluoridation of piped public water supplies in their areas, the amount of fluorine added not to exceed one part per million. The local sanitary authorities operating the water supplies are obliged to co-operate as agents of the health boards in fluoridation. The scheme was commenced in the Dublin area in 1964 and has by now been extended to most of the piped water supply schemes in the country. Fifty-six per cent of the population is now served by fluoridated water supplies (most of the remainder are in areas not served by piped supplies or in areas where the piped schemes are small and not suited to the installation of fluoridation equipment). Before fluoridation was introduced, detailed surveys were carried out on the incidence of dental caries in children. Studies are at present in progress to produce comparative figures of incidence in those areas where fluoridation has been in operation for some years. Preliminary results show a marked reduction in the incidence of caries after the introduction of fluoridation.

In some areas where there are not water supplies suitable for fluoridation, schemes have been brought in for applying fluoride by means of regular mouth-rinsing by the children, under suitable supervision.

Ophthalmic services
The health boards employ part-time ophthalmologists to examine eyes, to treat ailments and diseases and to prescribe spectacles. Spectacles are supplied by opticians under contract with the health boards. Hospital in-patient and out-patient care for the eyes is, of course, part of the general hospital care programme described in the next chapter.

Aural services
Consultant services for the treatment of ear defects are also part of the general hospital care programme. The community health services programme is concerned specifically with the assessment of hearing ability and the provision of hearing aids. Specially trained public health nurses carry out audiometry tests and the health boards have arrangements with the National Rehabilitation Board to provide hearing aids for those eligible for the service.

Community Welfare Programme

Welfare services are the responsibility of a number of Departments of State and of several subordinate authorities. However, because many aspects of welfare are closely linked with health care—particularly in relation to children and the aged—the health agencies have developed, and are continuing to develop, an increasing role in the provision of personal welfare services. This chapter deals only with the welfare services which come within the general scope of the health agencies. Specifically in the case of income maintenance services, those dealt with by the Department of Social Welfare are not covered except for the scheme of supplementary benefits which are administered by the health boards.[15]

Cash benefits
Maintenance allowances are paid by health boards to disabled persons over 16 years of age who are unable to provide for their own maintenance. The maximum rate for these allowances is fixed in regulations made by the Minister for Health (the maximum at present is £15.20 per week). These allowances are paid only to persons whose disability has lasted, or is expected to last, for one year from its onset. Those maintained in institutions are not eligible for the allowances. There were 24,862 beneficiaries under this scheme on 31 December 1976.

Health boards also pay maintenance allowances to persons receiving treatment for infectious diseases. Primarily, this scheme is applicable to those with tuberculosis, but it also covers those suffering from poliomyelitis, diphtheria, typhoid, paratyphoid, typhus, dysentery, salmonella infection, scarlet fever and streptococcal sore throat. The scheme is applicable to persons undergoing treatment to the satisfaction of the local medical officer who are unable to make 'reasonable and proper provision for their own maintenance or the maintenance of their dependants'. The scales of allowances are fixed by the Minister for Health and are varied from time to time in line with changes in allowances under Social Welfare schemes.

[15]The services of the Department of Social Welfare are described in 'Social Insurance and Social Assistance in Ireland', by D. Farley (Institute of Public Administration, Dublin 1968).

Allowances may also be paid to carriers of the diseases referred to above. If, through taking precautions against the spread of infection, a person is rendered incapable of carrying on his ordinary occupation and is thereby 'unable to make reasonable and proper provision for his own maintenance or the maintenance of his dependants', an allowance may be paid to him. A case in point would be a typhoid carrier employed in a restaurant who is directed to give up the handling of food.

Cash grants in respect of confinements are paid by health boards for women with full eligibility. The rate of the grant is £8 for each child. These grants are distinct from (and may be supplementary to) the maternity benefits given for insured persons under the Social Welfare Acts. Health boards also make arrangements for supplying milk or milk substitutes to expectant and nursing mothers with full eligibility and to children under five years of age 'whose parents are unable from their own resources to provide the children with an adequate supply of milk'.

Health boards also operate a scheme of cash payments to blind persons.

In 1973 a scheme was introduced for the payment of 'constant care' allowances to the parents of disabled children maintained at home. The rate of this allowance is at present £35 a month and it is paid irrespective of the means of the parents. Allowances were being paid for 4,044 children under this scheme on 31 December 1976.

The home assistance service which was the responsibility of local authorities and was under the general control of the Department of Social Welfare was replaced on 1 July 1977 by a new scheme of supplementary welfare allowances. This scheme is operated by the health boards but is governed by regulations made by the Minister for Social Welfare.

Home helps

The home assistance service had traditionally been used as an ancillary to the health services in the maintenance at home of the aged and of sick or infirm persons. More specific authority for this purpose was given to the health boards under the Health Act 1970 (Section 61). The boards were given a broad power to make arrangements for the maintenance at home of sick or infirm persons and certain other categories—with specific reference to cases which would otherwise need to be maintained in an institution. The health boards also have the power to give grants to voluntary agencies providing services 'similar or ancillary to' the services of the boards.[16] Under these provisions, health boards themselves employ home helps and make grants to voluntary agencies. They also make grants to voluntary agencies towards the cost of meals-on-wheels.

Care of children

Orphans and children who are deserted by their parents and who have no one else to look after them may be boarded-out by health boards.[17] A child whose parents cannot provide the necessities of life may also be boarded-out, with the agreement of the parents. The boarding-out arrangement normally lasts until sixteen years of age, but the health board may, after this age, continue boarding-out for the completion of a child's education. The regulations require that a contract be entered into between the board and the foster-parent and specify conditions as respects the suitability of the latter and certain facilities which must be available. Officers of the health board (generally social workers or public health nurses) and Department of Health inspectors may visit boarded-out children and the foster-homes.

Health boards may also pay for the keep of such children in 'approved schools'. These are industrial schools and orphanages, generally maintained by religious orders. The board may also arrange for the placing of a boarded-out child in 'any suitable trade calling or business'.

The total number of children in these categories under the care of health boards was 2,013 on 31 March, 1977.

The Children Acts, 1908 to 1957, are a comprehensive code for the protection of children against many forms of victimisation. Health boards are directly concerned only with the sections of the Acts which relate to the supervision of children placed in foster-homes, or placed in employment in certain circumstances.[18] The intention to receive a child under sixteen as

---

[16]Under section 65 of the Health Act, 1953.

[17]Sections 55 to 57 of the Health Act, 1953 and the Boarding-out of Children Regulations, 1954 govern this.

[18]Part I of the Children Act, 1908, as amended (mainly by section 57 of the Health Act, 1953 and sections 2 and 3 of the Children Act, 1957).

a foster-child for reward (or if the child is illegitimate, without reward) must be notified to the health board and the board has the responsibility to satisfy itself about the suitability of the home. It must arrange for the regular visiting of the child in the home.

Where any body or person, except a parent or other relative, proposes to send a child under eighteen years of age away for employment, the health board must also be notified and it has similar powers of supervision and visiting as respects that child. Health boards may contribute to the funds of any society for the prevention of cruelty to children.[19]

The legal adoption of children is provided for in the Adoption Act, 1952, which comes under the Minister for Justice. That Act established a body, An Bord Uchtála (the Adoption Board), with the function of approving of and registering adoptions. The Board itself does not arrange adoptions but registers societies with this as their object. Before registering an adoption, the Board satisfies itself as to the suitability of the adopters and may refuse an adoption order if it thinks fit. The effect of an adoption order is that a child acquires the surname of the adopters and, generally speaking, is placed in the same position as if he or she had been born legitimately to the adopters. Where a child boarded-out under the provisions described above is adopted by the foster-parents, the health board is no longer liable for its maintenance but, so that there would be no disincentive on the part of the foster-parents to adopt a child if they so wished, the health board is authorised to continue to contribute to the maintenance of the child as if still boarded-out.[20]

[19]Section 65(2) of Health Act, 1953.
[20]Section 55(9) of Health Act, 1953.

Chapter Eleven

The General Hospital Care Programme

The general hospital care programme is concerned broadly with that part of the health services in which care is provided for acute cases in or at hospitals. The programme does not, however, cover care for acute conditions at psychiatric hospitals. For budgetary purposes, the programme is divided as follows

regional hospitals (excluding voluntary)
public voluntary hospitals
health board county hospitals
private voluntary hospitals
district hospitals
health board long-stay hospitals
voluntary long-stay hospitals
ambulance services

The programme is the most expensive branch of the health services, absorbing 47 per cent of the non-capital expenditure and 59 per cent of the capital expenditure. The estimated current expenditure for 1978 on each of these categories is shown on page 182.

Eligibility for hospital services
For the treatment of the scheduled infectious diseases, which include tuberculosis (see pages 187 and 188) and for certain diseases and disabilities of a long-term nature in children, hospital care is available without a means test. Out-patient services are similarly available for defects noticed at child health examinations. Otherwise, the availability of in-patient and out-patient hospital services is governed by the conditions described in Chapter Eight.[1] There is no charge for the services made

[1]Article 12 of the Infectious Diseases Regulations, 1948, sections 52 and 56 of the Health Act, 1970 and articles 6 and 7 of the Health Services (Amendment) Regulations, 1971. The long-term conditions are: mental handicap, mental illness, phenylketonuria, cystic fibrosis, spina bifida, hydrocephalus, haemophilia, cerebral palsy, multiple sclerosis, muscular dystrophies, parkinsonism and acute leukaemia in children.

available by a health board where they are provided in a public ward in one of its own hospitals or in a hospital with which it has an arrangement. There are charges, however, for those who elect to go into private or semi-private accommodation. The position of these vis-à-vis voluntary health insurance is referred to on page 110.

A person not content to take what is offered by the health board may make his own arrangements to get like services in any hospital or nursing home on a list approved by the Minister. When a person does this, the health board is obliged to make a payment to the hospital or home on his behalf.[2] This payment is somewhat less than the cost to the health board if it had arranged itself for the services.

In the case of hospital treatment for injuries received in road traffic accidents, there is a special provision in the regulations absolving the health board from financial responsibility except where it is established to the satisfaction of its chief executive officer that the applicant for services was not getting damages from another person in respect of the injuries.[3] This restriction does not, of course, prevent a person receiving treatment. Generally, it will be long after treatment is completed when the issue of financial responsibility is cleared up.

The hospitals of Ireland

Two groups comprise the public hospital system of the country—the voluntary hospitals and the hospitals, formerly owned by the local authorities, which are now administered by the health boards.

Some public hospitals do not fall clearly into either of the two main categories. There are, in addition, a number of private hospitals not included in the public system.

The following table shows for each category the number of hospitals, the number of beds and the number of patients treated in 1976.[4]

The health board hospitals

On 1 April 1971, the health boards took over from the local

---

[2]Section 54 of Health Act, 1970.
[3]Article 6(3) of Health Services Regulations, 1971.
[4]The table is a digest of information in 'Statistical Information relevant to the Health Services, 1978' published by the Stationery Office.

Table 1—Hospitals, beds and patients in 1976

Type of Hospital	Number of hospitals	Number of beds	Average stay in days
Health Board Hospitals			
Regional	8	2,113	8.8
County	24	3.304	8.6
District	52	1,968	21.6
Fever	8	575	18.6
Orthopaedic	5	655	22.3
Total health board hospitals	97	8,615	10.9
Voluntary Public Hospitals			
General (Teaching)	16	4,181	11.8
General (Non-Teaching)	7	975	9.5
Maternity	5	934	6.9
Paediatric	4	747	8.9
Cancer	3	307	14.7
Eye and Ear	2	230	7.2
Orthopaedic	5	706	38.8
Cottage	5	136	27.2
Total voluntary public hospitals	47	8,216	10.7
Private Hospitals	16	1,558	not available
Total	160	18,389	10.8

authorities all the hospitals which were then in their charge. The origins of these hospitals are referred to in earlier chapters. They range from the few major teaching hospitals (the regional hospitals in Cork, Galway and Limerick) through the county hospitals described on pages 7 and 17 down to district

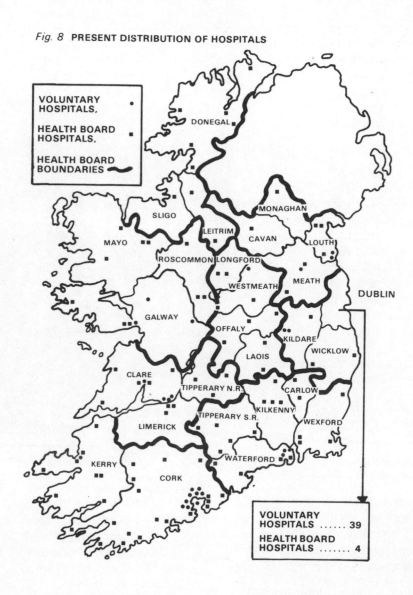

Fig. 8 **PRESENT DISTRIBUTION OF HOSPITALS**

hospitals, of which there are a number in most counties. The health board hospitals also include tuberculosis and other infectious diseases hospitals and orthopaedic hospitals. Most of the health board hospitals are relatively modern.

The law governing the provision and maintenance of hospitals by the health boards is contained in Part III of the Health Act, 1970, which gives a general authority for the provision and maintenance of hospitals and specifies the conditions under which changes can be made or institutions discontinued. The employment of staff for these hospitals is governed by the general provisions on officers and servants in health boards referred to in Chapter Six.

The standard pattern of staffing for the average county hospital at consultant level has been one surgeon and one physician, with services of a radiologist and an anaesthetist. For some of the hospitals, the pattern includes an obstetrician-gynaecologist and the medical staff in each case normally includes registrars and a number of house surgeons and physicians. The present policy on consultant staffing, as determined by Comhairle na nOspidéal, favours more than one of each class of consultant in each acute hospital and a number of the county hospitals are now so staffed.

The regional hospitals, each of which is, for specialities, a centre for a number of counties, are larger than the county hospitals and have greater numbers of consultant staff. All of the hospitals, of course, employ large numbers of nurses. The regional hospitals and a number of the county hospitals are nurse training schools.

The district hospitals are small institutions, generally ranging in size between twenty and forty beds. Each has the part-time services of a general practitioner, who acts as medical officer to the hospital. A small nursing staff is employed in each case. The services in these hospitals are limited to medical and, in some of them, to maternity cases requiring non-specialised care.

The expenses of running the health board hospitals are met from the board's budgets and thus come within the general financial provisions referred to in Chapter Seven.

The voluntary hospitals
The following extract from the report of the Consultative

Council on the General Hospital Services (the Fitzgerald Report) describes the development of the voluntary hospital system:

'1.2 The Irish voluntary hospital movement had its origins in the early decades of the 18th century and, because of the penal restrictions of the period on religious communities, was initially entirely lay in character. Philanthropic individuals, moved by the conditions of the sick poor, voluntarily took on themselves the task of establishing and running hospitals and raising money for them. It was a form of charity to the public not available in Ireland since the closure of the monasteries following the Reformation. On the other hand, in Britain, under Elizabethan legislation, a system of rate-supported public parochial assistance, including provision for the poor infirm, had been devised, but it had not been extended to Ireland.

1.3 The development of the Irish voluntary hospital was almost entirely confined to the city areas, particularly to Dublin. The movement depended largely for its support on the commercial and professional classes, an element not significantly represented in rural areas. Many of the hospitals had a short career, because of lack of continued financial support, but some of the earliest voluntary hospitals have survived to the present day. In Dublin, the Charitable Infirmary, Jervis Street; Dr. Steevens' Hospital; Mercer's Hospital; the Rotunda Maternity Hospital; the Royal Hospital for Incurables and the Meath Hospital all have early 18th century origins, and some of them were the earliest hospitals of their type in the world. The Dublin House of Industry, which eventually included in its complex of buildings the Richmond, Whitworth and Hardwicke Hospitals, started developing in 1773 and now forms St. Laurence's Hospital. The North Infirmary and the South Infirmary, Cork, also date from the same period as do, among others, the County and City Infirmary, Waterford.

1.4 During the first half of the 19th century the voluntary hospital movement was still the main force in providing for the sick poor. In Dublin, Sir Patrick Dun's Hospital, the Coombe Maternity Hospital, the Adelaide Hospital, the Royal City of Dublin Hospital, the Royal Victoria Eye and

Ear Hospital and the National Children's Hospital, Harcourt Street, came into existence. Barrington's Hospital was opened in Limerick. A significant influence on voluntary hospital development was the growth of more liberal political attitudes and the lifting of restrictions on the Catholic community, thus allowing the foundation of a number of new Irish Orders of Religious dedicated to the care of the sick poor. The Irish Sisters of Charity founded St. Vincent's Hospital, Dublin, in 1834. The Sisters of Mercy opened the Mercy Hospital in Cork in 1857 and the Mater Misericordiae Hospital in Dublin in 1861. A great expansion of these and other Orders, took place from then on, resulting in a most important contribution to the Irish hospital provision, among other examples of the charitable actions of these Orders.'

Most of the present-day voluntary hospitals are in Dublin, with smaller numbers in Cork and Limerick cities. The bases and management authorities for the hospitals vary widely. Some are owned and operated by religious orders, others are incorporated by charter or statute and work under lay boards of governors. Some, such as the North and South Infirmaries in Cork and the Meath Hospital, Dublin, are still tied in by statute with the public authorities. An important group of hospitals in Dublin are associated by the Hospitals Federation and Amalgamation Act, 1961, which was introduced by the Minister at their request. The initial object of this Act was to allow these hospitals to join in a federation, with the ultimate aim of their legal amalgamation. Similarly, five voluntary hospitals in Cork have combined under the Cork Voluntary Hospitals Board, established in 1977.[5]

All but a minor part of the current expenditure of the voluntary hospitals is now met by public funds, as is shown by the figures for the year ended 31 December 1977.

Other public hospitals
There are a number of specially set up hospital authorities which cut across the broad division of the hospital system referred to above. St. Laurence's Hospital, Dublin, for

[5]Under the Cork Voluntary Hospitals Board (Establishment) Order, 1977.

Table 2—Source of voluntary hospital funds

Source	£ million
Met from public funds	71.0
Met from other sources	10.3
Total	81.3

example, is controlled by a statutory board, the members of which are appointed by the Minister.[6] Five bodies established under the Health (Corporate Bodies) Act, 1961, are concerned with the administration of specific hospitals. One, the St. Luke's Hospital Board, provides a cancer service: the members of this board are appointed by the Minister. Another, the National Rehabilitation Board, is concerned jointly with the Sisters of Mercy in the operation of the National Medical Rehabilitation Centre, at Dun Laoghaire. The Cork Hospitals Board was charged with the building of a new hospital at Cork (but the hospital, having been commissioned, is managed by the Southern Health Board). The St. James's Hospital Board, with members appointed by the Eastern Health Board and the Federation of Dublin Voluntary Hospitals, has taken over the management of the former St. Kevin's Hospital in Dublin, with a view to its joint development. The James Connolly Memorial Hospital Board, a similar body, which is representative of the Eastern Health Board and the Mater Misericordiae, St. Laurence's and Jervis Street Hospitals, was set up to develop general hospital facilities at the regional sanatorium at Blanchardstown, County Dublin.

Current developments in the Dublin area will affect a number of the voluntary and other hospitals. A new hospital being built at Beaumont on the north side of the city will replace Jervis Street and St. Laurence's Hospitals. The commissioning of the new St. James's hospital and the provision of a new hospital at Tallaght will lead to the closure of most of the older voluntary hospitals on the south side of the city.

Joint services
A nation-wide blood transfusion service, including the process-

[6]Under the St. Laurence's Hospital Act, 1943.

ing and supply of blood derivatives and blood products, is provided for the various hospitals by the Blood Transfusion Service Board. This is a board of twelve members appointed by the Minister.[7] Donation of blood is organised by the Board on a voluntary basis and its running expenses are met by contributions from the hospitals for the blood supplied.

The Hospitals Joint Services Board provides a service for the supply of sterile requisites to hospitals[8] and has also established a laundry to provide a centralised service for the Dublin hospitals. The Board has fifteen members who are appointed by the Minister.

Ambulance services

The health boards have taken over the operation of ambulance services formerly provided by the local health authorities. The boards have a general power to provide ambulances or other means of transport for the conveyance of patients.[9] In some areas, the fire brigades operate the ambulance service as agents of the health boards. Where necessary, Army helicopters are used, on a repayment basis, to convey patients.

The Fitzgerald Report

The Report of the Consultative Council on the General Hospital Services (the Fitzgerald Report) has, since it was published in 1968, provided a focus for discussion on the future development of the general hospital services. The report was prepared by a broadly representative group of consultants, under the chairmanship of the late Professor Patrick Fitzgerald, who were appointed as a consultative council by the Minister. The Council made important recommendations in relation to administration (these are referred to on page 34), but the essential part of its task was to report on the organisation and location of these services 'so as to secure, with due regard to the national resources, that the public is provided in a most effective way with the best possible services'.

[7] See the Blood Transfusion Service Board (Establishment) Order, 1965.
[8] See the Hospitals Sterile Supplies Board (Establishment) Order, 1965 as amended by another order in the same year.
[9] Section 57 of Health Act, 1970.

Having surveyed the present pattern of hospital services, the Council concluded that radical changes were necessary, involving a departure from many long-established concepts in regard to organisation, staffing and operation. Its recommendations on administration, involving the creation of a central 'consultants establishment board', regional hospital boards and hospital management committees, were aimed at achieving a reorganisation of the services involving closer co-ordination between the voluntary hospitals and the then local authority hospitals.

At the top level of the integrated structure, the Council recommended that there should be four regional hospitals, two in Dublin and one each in Cork and Galway. Each of these would provide a general service for its own hinterland and more specialised services for a wider area. The Council recommended that in nine other centres there should be general hospitals, each having at least 300 beds. The basic services provided in these would be general medicine, general surgery, obstetrics, gynaecology, pathology and radiology. In making this recommendation, the Council pointed to the advantages of larger units (which allow for more specialisation), better staffing arrangements (because of there being a number of physicians and surgeons attached to the hospital) and the better equipment which would be possible in such hospitals.

Each of the general hospitals recommended by the Council would serve a population of about 120,000 people. Only some of the county hospitals could be developed into these general hospitals and the functions of the others would change. The Council envisaged that these would take patients of family doctors, who could continue to care for them while in hospital, and would be backed by diagnostic facilities and a comprehensive consultant out-patient organisation. These centres, the Council pointed out, would have an important role in the care of long-stay geriatric patients. The district hospitals would also be used in conjunction with the family doctor service, but would not be regarded as having a role in the provision of acute care hospital services. In their development of these recommendations, the Council set out detailed proposals for their application throughout the country.

The Minister for Health announced acceptance of the

general principles of the Fitzgerald Report, but not of all the specific recommendations on the application of these principles throughout the country. The principles of the Report are reflected in the actions taken in Dublin since it was published and in developments in many other areas, but its specific recommendations for the county hospitals have not all been accepted.

Chapter Twelve

Special Hospital Care Programmes

The objective of the special hospital care programmes is to provide the diagnosis, care and treatment that will enable the mentally ill, the mentally handicapped and the old to enjoy a reasonable life and, where possible to return to the community.

Mental Health

Earlier chapters described the separate origins of the services for the mentally ill and the long-term convergence of these services and the general health services into the same administrative structure. This is now complete, as the health boards have, in each area, full responsibility for the mental health service. In its nature too, the mental health service has tended towards becoming more like the general health services, although the facilities for the psychiatric service are still mainly based on the nineteenth-century hospitals within which it developed.

Eligibility for mental hospital services
The rules on eligibility for care in and at psychiatric hospitals are on the whole the same as for general hospitals. For children under sixteen years of age, the full range of services is, however, available irrespective of their own or their parents' means.[1] Health boards make payments, as in the case of general hospital care, for persons going to private mental hospitals or homes for in-patient treatment.

Reception and maintenance of patients
The Mental Treatment Act, 1945, which is the basic statute on the mental health service, specifies three categories of patients in mental hospitals,—voluntary patients, temporary patients and those certified as 'persons of unsound mind'. Details of admission for each class are specified in the Act, which also details the procedures and restrictions in relation to the detention of patients and the patients' rights of appeal in relation to detention. A short summary of these provisions is given in Appendix H.

[1]See footnote 1, Chapter 11.

Admissions to mental hospitals in recent years have been mainly on a voluntary or temporary basis. Voluntary patients account for over three-quarters of the admissions and temporary patients for one-fifth: only 2 per cent of the total are admissions as 'persons of unsound mind.' There has been a steady fall in the total number of in-patients in the health boards' mental hospitals. In 1958 it was 21,075, in 1965 it was 18,642, in 1970 it was 15,392 and on 31 December 1977 it was 13,288. On the other hand, attendances at out-patient clinics have increased steadily.

There are twelve private mental hospitals. There is increasing co-operation between these and the health boards in providing services. There are about 1,000 places in these hospitals. The largest is St. Patrick's Hospital, Dublin, which had 398 in-patients on 31 December 1977.

Central Mental Hospital
The Central Mental Hospital, Dundrum, Dublin, the institution specially established in the nineteenth century for the reception of 'criminal lunatics', became the responsibility of the Eastern Health Board in September 1971. The admission of patients to this hospital is dealt with in Appendix H.

Commission of Inquiry on Mental Illness
The Commission of Inquiry on Mental Illness was appointed by the Minister for Health in 1961 to examine and report on the health services available for the mentally ill and on changes thought necessary or desirable in legislation. It reported in 1966, making wide-ranging recommendations.
The Commission—
  emphasised the need for active and early treatment of mental illness and for the integration of psychiatry and general medicine, and thus favoured a concept of psychiatric units in, or associated with, general hospitals;

  for long-stay patients, recommended that mental hospitals should be regarded not merely as centres for custodial care, but that planned and purposeful activity for the patients should be featured, with a view to their rehabilitation and restoration to the community as far as possible;

thought that the aim should be to have the number of long-stay places halved in fifteen years;

recommended that private psychiatric hospitals should, like the voluntary general hospitals, be involved in providing services for the health authorities;

stressed the need to give priority to the development of out-patient services;

thought that general practitioners should be encouraged to take a greater interest and a more active role in psychiatry and that public health personnel should play a greater part than heretofore in the promotion of mental health;

made specific recommendations on the problems of children, adolescents and the aged and on alcoholism, drug addiction, epilepsy and other special classes such as homicidal patients, psychopaths and sexual deviates;

advocated improved measures for prevention and research and for the education and training of professional staff and others in relation to psychiatry;

emphasised the need for more time being given to the study of psychiatry in the curricula of the medical schools;

recommended a number of amendments in the legislation dealing with the mentally ill, mainly designed towards making the reception and detention of most psychiatric patients more informal; and

recommended more flexible provisions in relation to the boarding-out of patients.

The recommendations of the Commission have largely been followed in the development of policy on the psychiatric services since it reported. Its recommendations were implemented, for example, in the transfer of the responsibility for the Central Mental Hospital to the Eastern Health Board and in the co-ordination with the private psychiatric hospitals in the Dublin area.

Mental Handicap

The identification and care of the mentally handicapped is divided between the community health services and the mentally handicapped programmes of the health boards. For institutional maintenance, reliance is placed mainly on voluntary homes, which receive payments on behalf of the health boards.

Eligibility for services
The normal rules for entitlement to hospital services nominally apply in relation to eligibility for the care of the mentally handicapped, but the care of all children up to the age of sixteen is free without reference to the parents' means.[2] As those over sixteen would have their income assessed in their own right, without reference to that of the parents or other relatives, it will be clear that very few mentally handicapped persons are in Category 3 and thus outside the scope of entitlement to the full range of the services.

Institutional care
A number of mentally handicapped, mainly adults, are in the district mental hospitals and other institutions of the health boards (the figure for these in 1974 was about 3,500). Special homes for the mentally handicapped are provided and administered by voluntary bodies, mainly religious Orders. In this field, the Brothers of Charity, the Daughters of Charity and the Hospitaller Order of St. John of God are the most prominent. Capital works are financed mainly by way of grants from the Hospitals Trust Fund.

A major part of the building programme for some years past has been directed towards adding to the number of places in residential centres available for the mentally handicapped. At the end of 1964, the total number of places available in such centres was 3,101. At the end of 1970, it had increased to 4,148 and by the end of 1976, it was 4,751. Further work in progress or planning will provide 1,369 more places.

[2] See footnote 2, Chapter 11.

Day centres are provided by a wide variety of voluntary bodies. The numbers attending these has increased very considerably in recent years.

Table 1 shows the numbers of mentally handicapped catered for by residential and non-residential centres and services on 31 December 1976.[3]

Table 1: Mentally handicapped in residential and day care centres.

Type of Centre or Service	Numbers catered for		Total
	Under 16 years	Over 16 years	
Residential centres of voluntary bodies	2,198	2,287	4,485
Residential centres of health boards	205	61	266
Hostels and lodgings	128	106	234
Total residential	2,531	2,454	4,985
Day schools and classes	4,088	484	4,572
Day care	614	161	775
Day workshops and occupational centres	11	560	571
Total day care	4,713	1,205	5,918
Grand total	7,244	3,659	10,903

The Aged

The care of the aged is not a monopoly of any one part of the health services. Those old people who are living at home have available to them the range of services referred to earlier, subject to the general rules about eligibility and they similarly have access to the acute general hospital services. Many aged people,

[3]More detailed statistics are given in 'Statistical Information relevant to the Health Service, 1978', published by the Stationery Office.

however, reach the stage when they can no longer be looked after in a private dwelling and must be taken into a home. For such of these as are unable to arrange this from their own resources, the health boards provide maintenance.

Traditionally, the institutional care of the aged was provided in the county homes which were adapted from some of the nineteenth-century workhouses. The Inter-Departmental Committee on the Care of the Aged, which reported in 1968, recommended that the concept of these homes should be abandoned and that a system should be developed under which the need of the aged for institutional care would be carefully assessed, steps would be taken to assign patients to the most appropriate form of care and every effort would be made to rehabilitate patients and restore them to the community. The Committee recommended that provision for the aged should be made in four main types of accommodation— general hospitals, geriatric assessment units, long-stay hospital units and welfare homes. These recommendations form the basis of current policy on development of the services. It is recognised, however, that development must start from the existing facilities as there is no single plan which can be imposed throughout the country. The planning of the special new assessment centres is proceeding in a number of centres and new small welfare homes are being provided.

At the end of 1975, there were 46 geriatric hospitals, with 8,411 patients, 23 welfare homes, with 896 residents and 3,681 were accommodated in 108 voluntary and private institutions. In all, there were 177 institutions, with 12,988 residents.

Chapter Thirteen

Vital Statistics and Research

Information on the size of the population, on birth, death and marriage rates and on the numbers affected by different diseases and injuries is vital to the organisation of the health services. This information is necessary in identifying problems, in designing services, in deciding on priorities in development and in evaluating the results of action taken. The reports prepared by the Central Statistics Office on the periodic census of population form the basis for statistical information on the health services. These give to the Department and to the health boards information on the numbers for whom health services must be designed. To build on this, the Department and other agencies analyse information specifically relating to health and the services.

Births, deaths and marriages
Under the Minister for Health, an tArd Chláraitheoir (the Registrar-General) has the responsibility for organising the registration of births, deaths and marriages. He operates through local registrars who come under the general supervision of the health boards. As well as the basic data needed for registration, there is compiled, through the registration system, further detailed information relating to births and deaths. From this, annual reports on vital statistics are published by the Minister, with the co-operation of the Central Statistics Office. The detailed operation of this system is described in Appendix I. Some graphs illustrating results obtained from analysing these statistics are shown at the end of this chapter. They are reproduced from the Report on Vital Statistics, 1974, by courtesy of the Minister for Health and the Controller of the Stationery Office.

The registration system is concerned with the causes of death but not with the incidence of disease in living persons. The only formal requirements for providing information relating to this are in the requirements to notify infectious diseases referred to in Chapter Ten.

150

The Medical Research Council
The Medical Research Council was incorporated as a limited liability company in 1937, with the object of organising and carrying out research in medicine. The Council has nine members, made up of eight nominees of the Universities and other medical licensing bodies and a chairman appointed by the Minister. The Council administers funds made available to it by the Minister and from other sources. Its total budget for 1978 was £375,000.

The Council's primary concern is with basic research on the causes of and cures for diseases and most of its funds are devoted to giving grants for projects in these fields. It has not been part of the Council's function to conduct widespread projects on morbidity or on the operation of the health services.

The Medico-Social Research Board
To extend work on morbidity, the Medico-Social Research Board was established in 1965.[1] Its functions are to organise and administer surveys and statistical research in relation to the incidence of human diseases, injuries, deformities and defects, and the operation of the health services. The Board has fourteen members who are appointed by the Minister.

The Board conducts a survey in relation to in-patients in general hospitals. The hospitals are asked to complete statistical summaries for all patients and to send them to the Board, which has the data processed by computer. The information which this survey is producing includes a diagnostic index for each of the participating hospitals and for each participating consultant (on request), and national statistics, showing discharges from hospitals by reference to diagnosis and duration of stay. Relevant statistics are given for the separate health board areas. By 1977, the number of hospitals participating in the survey was 59, from which there are about 220,000 discharges a year.

A national psychiatric in-patient reporting system is also operated by the Board and studies have been undertaken by it on specific psychiatric questions. It has also conducted a census of mentally handicapped in the community and in institutions. Follow-up studies on the causes of mental handicap and its

[1]By the Medico-Social Research Board (Establishment) Order, 1965.

prevalence are being undertaken. A study of peri-natal and child mortality and morbidity in Ireland is being initiated by the Board and among other studies which it has completed are one into the incidence of ischaemic heart disease and one into the incidence of strokes (both of these were carried out in collaboration with the World Health Organisation). A study on air pollution as part of the EEC studies on environmental control has also been completed.

Future needs

The future decision-making processes of all involved in the health services in Ireland will call for more information on which to frame policies and take decisions. Good planning and execution of policy always calls for plenty of hard facts and figures and the planning systems in the Department and the health boards, to operate at all, must be fed an adequate diet of statistics. The Department, the registration authorities, the Medico-Social Research Board, the hospital co-ordinating bodies and the health boards will all be involved in this.

Each year the Planning Unit of the Department issues a volume giving a digest of statistical material relevant to the health services. This is derived from the sources mentioned above and other sources.[2]

[2]These volumes may be purchased from the Government Publications Sales Office, GPO Arcade, Dublin 1.

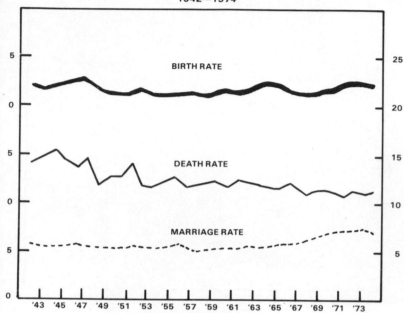

Fig. 9 BIRTH, MARRIAGE AND DEATH RATES (PER 1,000 POPULATION)
1942—1974

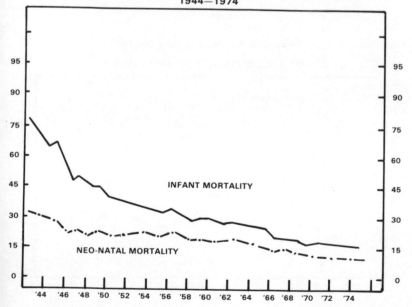

Fig. 10 INFANT AND NEO-NATAL MORTALITY (PER 1,000 LIVE BIRTHS)
1944—1974

Fig. 11 DEATH RATES (PER 1,000 POPULATION) FROM TUBERCULOSIS &
CANCER 1945—1974

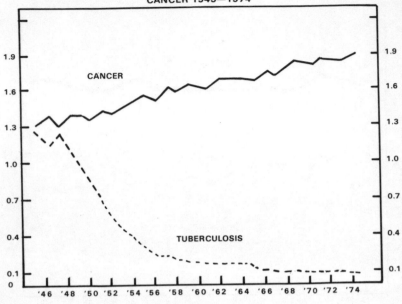

DEATH RATES FROM LUNG CANCER

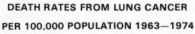

Fig. 12   PER 100,000 POPULATION 1963—1974

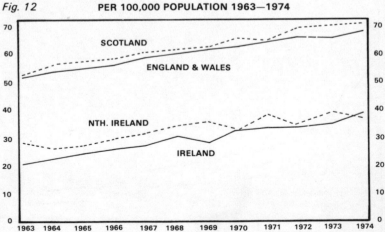

Official Organisations Concerned with Health Services

This list includes only those administrative organisations appointed by statute or by the Minister under statute. Particulars of many other organisations, including representative professional bodies may be found in the *Administration Yearbook and Diary* (published by the Institute of Public Administration). Particulars of the voluntary hospitals are given in the *Irish Medical and Hospitals Directory* (published by General Publications Ltd., 59 Merrion Square).

Central and Regional
Department of Health, Custom House, Dublin 1.
Comhairle na nOspidéal, Corrigan House, Fenian St.,
    Dublin 2.
Dublin Regional Hospitals Board, Corrigan House, Fenian
    St., Dublin 2.
Cork Regional Hospitals Board, Corrigan House, Fenian St.,
    Dublin 2.
Galway Regional Hospitals Board, Merlin Park, Galway.

Standing Central Advisory Bodies
National Health Council, Custom House, Dublin 1.
Comhairle na Nimheanna, Custom House, Dublin 1.
Therapeutic Substances Advisory Committee, Custom House,
    Dublin 1.
Food Advisory Committee, Custom House, Dublin 1.

Executive Agencies

Health Boards
Eastern Health Board, 1 James St., Dublin 8.
Midland Health Board, Arden Road, Tullamore, Co. Offaly.
Mid-Western Health Board, 31/33 Catherine St., Limerick.
North-Eastern Health Board, Ceanannus Mór, Co. Meath.

North-Western Health Board, Manorhamilton, Co. Leitrim.
South-Eastern Health Board, Arus Sláinte, Patrick St.,
 Kilkenny.
Southern Health Board, Cork Farm Centre, Dennehy's
 Cross, Cork.
Western Health Board, Merlin Park, Galway.

Statutory Bodies
Hospitals Trust Board, Bank of Ireland, Head Office, Lr.
 Baggot St., Dublin 2.
St. Laurence's Hospital Board, North Brunswick St.,
 Dublin 7.
Voluntary Health Insurance Board, 20/23 Lr. Abbey St.,
 Dublin 1.

Bodies under Health (Corporate Bodies) Act, 1961
Blood Transfusion Service Board, Pelican House, Lr. Leeson
 St., Dublin 2.
Cork Hospitals Board, c/o St. Finbarr's Hospital, Cork.
Dublin Dental Hospital Board, 20 Lincoln Place, Dublin 2.
Hospital Joint Services Board, Holylands, Grange Road,
 Rathfarnham, Dublin 14.
James Connolly (Memorial) Hospital Board, Blanchardstown,
 Co. Dublin.
Medico-Social Research Board, 73 Lr. Baggot St., Dublin 2.
National Drugs Advisory Board, Charles Lucas House, 57C
 Harcourt St., Dublin 2.
National Rehabilitation Board, 25 Clyde Road, Dublin 4.
St. Luke's Hospital Board, Highfield Road, Rathgar,
 Dublin 6.
St. James's Hospital Board, James's St., Dublin 8.
Hospital Bodies Administrative Bureau, Corrigan House,
 Fenian St., Dublin 2.
The Health Education Bureau, 52 Upr. Mount St., Dublin 2.
Beaumont Hospital Board, 52 Upr. Mount St., Dublin 2.
The Cork Voluntary Hospitals Board, c/o South Infirmary
 Hospital, Cork.

Other Executive Bodies
Health Inspectors' Training Board, Hawkins House, Dublin 2.

Medical Research Council of Ireland, 9 Clyde Road, Dublin 4.

Registration Bodies
An Bord Altranais (Nursing Board), 11 Fitzwilliam Place,
 Dublin 2.
Bord na Radharcmhastóirí (Opticians Board), 18 Fitzwilliam
 Square, Dublin 2.
Dental Board, 57 Merrion Square, Dublin 2.
Medical Registration Council, 6 Kildare St., Dublin 2.
Pharmaceutical Society of Ireland, 18 Shrewsbury Road,
 Dublin 4.

APPENDIX B

Officers and Servants of Health Boards

The following are the directions which have been issued by the Minister for Health to health boards in relation to the appointment and conditions of service of officers and servants employed by health boards.

Introduction
1. Reference throughout the directions to the transfer of staff are to the transfer directed under the provisions of Sections 34, 35 and 37 of the Health Act, 1970, and references to transferred staff are to staff so transferred.

Section 14

Determination of the number and type of appointments
2. Where a health board makes a determination in respect of the number and type of appointments to be made it shall be on the basis that no appointments of officers will be made in respect of such determination until the Minister consents except:
(a) insofar as the appointments may be required to maintain the staffing of institutions and outdoor services at the levels which obtained under the health authorities involved in the transfer of staff immediately prior to such transfer;
(b) insofar as the determination relates to additional appointments of a temporary nature which the chief executive officer considers urgently necessary and which are made for a period not exceeding four weeks and
(c) in such other cases as the Minister may direct.

Selection procedure other than through the Local Appointments Commission
3. The chief executive officer shall comply with the following provisions when making an appointment as an officer to which the Local Authorities (Officers and Employees) Acts, 1926 and 1940 do not apply.

158

(a) As soon as possible after the occurrence of a vacancy an advertisement shall be published in the public press inviting applications from qualified persons and specifying a closing date which allows a reasonable period for potential candidates to inform themselves of the particulars of the appointment and to apply in such form as may be required. If it is intended to make more than one appointment, the advertisement should so indicate. If a panel is to be formed from which further appointments may be made if required during a period ahead, it should be so stated in the advertisement.

(b) The selection of a candidate or candidates to be appointed or of the candidates to be placed in order of merit on a panel shall be by means of a selection procedure appropriate to the appointment having regard to the nature of the duties, the knowledge and experience necessary for the efficient performance of the duties and the qualifications for the appointment. Where the selection is not made on the results of a competitive examination, whether a general examination conducted by the Department of Education or an examination held specially on behalf of the health board, a suitably constituted interview board should be set up to assess the relative merits of candidates. A short list of candidates to attend before the interview board may be prepared by the latter from an examination of statements of qualifications furnished by candidates, at the request of the chief executive officer if he is satisfied that this course is justified, provided that the remaining candidates who possess the essential qualifications are notified accordingly.

(c) Subject to paragraphs 4, 8(c) and 18 appointments should be made by the chief executive officer in accordance with the results of the competitive examination or the recommendations of the interview board, except where it is necessary for him, on the grounds of character, health, or previous employment record, to decide that a particular candidate is not suitable for employment. The chief executive officer should satisfy himself on these points by having a medical examination carried out and by making appropriate enquiries.

Preferences for knowledge of Irish Language
4. (a) In making appointments a chief executive officer shall have regard to the provisions of the Local Officers (Irish

Language) Regulations, 1966 relating to the grant of preference for a knowledge of the Irish language as if health boards were local authorities.

(b) It is recommended that in the selection of candidates for appointments other than appointments in which preferences are granted as at sub-paragraph (c) and (d), extra marks be granted to candidates in respect of their knowledge of Irish on the basis of a percentage of the marks allotted by the interview board in the assessment of their relative merits, at the rate of 6% to candidates adjudged to possess a competent knowledge of Irish and at the rate of 3% in the case of candidates adjudged to possess a good knowledge of Irish.

(c) For appointments as assistant county medical officer or equivalent grades, dental surgeon and public health nurse the preferences recommended, in view of their duties in relation to school-children, are that

(i) the best qualified candidate from amongst those who possess a competent knowledge of Irish will be selected provided he or she is otherwise suitable;

(ii) if no qualified and suitable candidate possessing a competent knowledge of Irish is available additional marks will be given for a good knowledge of Irish and subject to this the best qualified candidate will be selected provided he or she is otherwise suitable;

(d) For the appointments mentioned at sub-paragraph (c) and any other appointment, if the duties are to be performed in a Gaeltacht district, the preference set out at sub-paragraph (c) should be extended as follows:

(i) the best qualified candidate from amongst those who possess a competent knowledge of Irish will be selected provided he or she is otherwise suitable;

(ii) if no qualified and suitable candidate possessing a competent knowledge of Irish is available, the best qualified candidate from amongst those who possess a good knowledge of Irish will be selected, provided he or she is otherwise suitable;

(iii) if no qualified and suitable candidate with a good knowledge of Irish is available, the best qualified candidate will be selected, provided he or she is otherwise suitable.

[These provisions are under review. As the first part of this review the following amendments have been made:

(a) For the purpose of special competitive written examinations or competitions based on Department of Education examination results (i.e. mainly for school leavers) candidates will, in addition to whatever other essential subjects are prescribed in the marking scheme for any particular grade, be required to qualify in either the subject Irish or the subject English and if a candidate qualifies in both Irish and English the marks received for both will be aggregated to the marks received for the other essential subjects, and

(b) If in addition to written examinations candidates are interviewed for the purpose of selection candidates will have the option of being interviewed in Irish or English.]

Panels

5. (a) Where appointments in a particular grade are made frequently and a panel is formed for such appointments in accordance with the provisions of paragraphs 3(a) and (b), either the number of names entered on the panel should be limited to the number of appointments which can be expected with reasonable certainty to be made within a year from the setting up of the panel or, if it is expedient to place a greater number of names on the panel to allow for wastage or for other reasons, the duration of the panel when it is being formed should be expressly limited to a specified period. Normally this period would be one year but it should not exceed two years.

(b) The chief executive officer may continue to draw on panels formed by local authorities involved in the transfer of staff to the board which were still in existence immediately prior to the transfer on the conditions which applied to the panels when formed by local authorities.

(c) Where a panel for the appointment of clerical officers or clerk-typists has been created and has expired and a new panel has not yet been created, the chief executive officer may appoint to a vacant office of clerical officer or clerk-typist a permanent officer of equivalent rank who is in the employment of another health board or local authority, subject to the consent of the health board or local authority concerned.

Appointments to which normal selection procedure need not be applied

6. Apart from the chief executive officer responsibility to decide the suitability for appointment of every person appointed, the provisions of paragraph 3 need not be applied to appointments referred to at (a) to (c) and in the circumstances referred to at (d) to the extent shown:

(a) Additional temporary appointments of the type referred to at paragraph 2(b).

(b) (i) Additional appointments of a temporary nature which are being made in compliance with paragraph 2, other than those referred to at 2(b), and

(ii) temporary appointments as substitutes for permanent officers in place of permanent appointments pending the making of the latter, if they are urgently necessary or, if the chief executive officer is satisfied that advertisement would not be warranted because of the short duration of the temporary appointment or that advertisement would be unlikely to attract any other applicants. (As a normal rule, temporary appointments pending the making of permanent appointments on the recommendation of the Local Appointments Commissioners should be made following advertisement).

(c) The appointment as an officer in a hospital of a person who is a member of a religious order which is associated with the administration of that hospital in replacement of another member of that order who had been appointed without advertisement or competition.

(d) Where the Minister consents that a particular appointment or appointments of a particular class may be made from among permanent officers of the health board or of health boards generally through a special selection procedure such appointments may be made without reference to paragraph 4 (a) and (b).

Informing Appointees of the Conditions of Appointment

7. (a) When making an appointment the chief executive officer should ensure that the person to be appointed is made aware of the conditions on which the appointment is being made, including the conditions relating to the determination of duties,

the relevant qualifications for continuing as an officer, and the provisions relating to tenure of office in paragraph 8 and that he signs a form of acceptance of the appointment on such conditions.

(b) In the case of a temporary appointment the nature of it should be clearly specified in the conditions on which it is made. Apart from the special case of appointments of the type referred to at paragraph 2(b), a maximum period, which should in no case exceed 12 months, should be specified for each temporary appointment but an alternative period, if shorter, should also be specified in each case according to the circumstances e.g. (i) until a specified work or duty is completed in the case of an additional temporary appointment, (ii) until a permanent appointment is made where the temporary appointment is made in place of a permanent appointment pending the making of the latter or (iii) where the temporary appointment is that of substitute for an absent officer until the return of the officer to duty.

Tenure of Office

8. (a) Any permanent officer who ceases to be qualified to continue as an officer by reference to any of the qualifications approved of or directed by the Minister for his continuing as an officer shall on so ceasing to qualify cease to hold office.

(b) Any permanent officer who is required by the terms of his appointment to comply with specified requirements or conditions (including a requirement or condition that he shall acquire a specified qualification) before the expiration of a specified period shall cease to hold office at the end of such period unless within that period he has complied with such requirements or conditions.

(c) No person who already holds a permanent appointment under a health board or local authority shall be given another permanent appointment unless he ceases to hold his earlier appointment or unless the Minister's consent is given to his holding both appointments, and any permanent officer who obtains another permanent appointment under a health board or local authority shall cease to hold his existing appointment, unless the Minister has consented to his holding both appointments.

(d) Every permanent appointment of a person who is not already a permanent officer of a health board or of a local authority shall be made subject to the conditions that:

(i) the person appointed shall hold office for a probationary period of twelve months which the chief executive officer may at his discretion extend and

(ii) the person appointed shall cease to hold office at the end of his probationary period unless during such period the chief executive officer has certified that the service of such person is satisfactory.

(e) Every permanent appointment of a person who is already a permanent officer of a health board or of a local authority and who is already serving a probationary period shall be made subject to the conditions that:

(i) the person appointed shall hold office for a probationary period of such duration as with the probationary period served by the officer under the other health board or local authority shall be not less than twelve months which the chief executive officer may at his discretion extend and

(ii) the person appointed shall cease to hold office at the end of his probationary period unless during such period the chief executive officer has certified that the service of such person is satisfactory.

Granting of Sick Leave

9. (i) A chief executive officer may grant sick leave to an officer who is incapable of performing his duties owing to illness or physical injury if, and only if, the chief executive officer is satisfied that there is a reasonable expectation that such officer will be able to resume the performance of his duties and, in the case of a temporary officer, will be able to resume during his period of office.

(ii) The chief executive officer may require an officer to submit himself to independent medical examination before he is granted sick leave and at any time during the continuance of sick leave granted to him.

(iii) The chief executive officer may pay salary during sick leave to permanent officers in accordance with the following provisions:

(a) Except in the case mentioned in sub-paragraph (d) no

salary shall be paid to an officer when the sick leave granted to such an officer during any continuous period of four years exceeds in the aggregate 365 days.

(b) Subject to limitation mentioned in sub-paragraph (a), salary may be paid to an officer at the full rate in respect of any days sick leave unless, by reason of such payment the period of sick leave during which such officer has been paid full salary would exceed 183 days during the twelve months ending on such day.

(c) Subject to the limitation mentioned in sub-paragraph (a) salary may be paid at half the full rate after salary has ceased by reason of the provision in sub-paragraph (b) to be paid at the full rate.

(d) If before the payment of salary ceases by reason of the provision in sub-paragraph (a) the Minister so consents, salary may be paid to a pensionable officer with not less than ten years service notwithstanding the said sub-paragraph (a) at either half the full rate or at a rate estimated to be the rate of pension to which such officer would be entitled on retirement, whichever of such rates shall be the lesser.

(e) For the purposes of these provisions every day occurring within a continuous period of sick leave shall be reckoned as part of such period.

(iv) From the salary paid during sick leave to an officer who is an insured person within the meaning of the Social Welfare Acts, 1952 to 1968, there shall be deducted the amount of any payments to which such officer has become entitled under those Acts during the period of such sick leave.

(v) The chief executive officer may make appropriate salary payments during sick leave to a temporary officer if he considers that having regard to all the circumstances of the case, such payment is reasonable.

(vi) Where a permanent officer is suffering from tuberculosis and is undergoing treatment, the chief executive officer may extend the foregoing provisions to allow the payment of salary at three-quarters the full rate to the officer for the second six months of his illness and at half the full rate during the third six months of his illness.

Granting of leave other than sick leave

10. (1) The following provisions shall apply to the grant of leave other than sick leave to officers of health boards:

(a) in the local financial year during the whole of which an officer holds office, he shall be entitled to the number of days annual leave specified for his office;

(b) in a local financial year during part only of which he holds office he shall be entitled to a proportionately reduced number of days annual leave;

(c) if an officer transferred from a health authority to a health board was entitled as part of his conditions of service to a number of days annual leave greater than the number referred to in paragraph (a) or paragraph (b), as the case may be, he shall continue to be so entitled.

(2) The granting of leave other than sick leave to a temporary officer shall be at the discretion of the chief executive officer subject to the provisions set out in this direction in relation to permanent officers.

(3) (a) Special leave with pay may be granted by chief executive officers in the circumstances and on the conditions set out in the addendum. Where it is proposed, however, to grant special leave with pay other than for the purposes set out in the addendum the prior consent of the Minister must be obtained.

(b) Special leave without pay may be granted by the chief executive officer without reference to the Department, Officers applying for special leave without pay should be informed that any period of such special leave cannot be reckoned as service for the purposes of the Local Government Superannuation Act, 1956.

(c) Special leave without pay for a period exceeding 28 days should not be reckoned for the purposes of annual leave or increment. Special leave without pay granted for the following purposes may, however, be reckoned as service for incremental purposes:

(i) to general trained nurses to obtain a midwifery qualification;

(ii) to psychiatric nurses to obtain a general nursing qualification;

(iii) to general trained nurses to obtain a psychiatric nursing qualification;

(iv) to general trained or psychiatric nurses to obtain a qualification in nursing the mentally handicapped.

The grant of incremental credit for such periods should be conditional on the chief executive officer being satisfied that the officer concerned has endeavoured to the best of his ability to acquire the additional qualification without any avoidable loss of time.

(4) An officer shall not be granted leave other than sick leave save in accordance with these provisions.

Determination of Duties of Officers

11. (a) Where duties of transferred officers have not been determined in accordance with the directions of the Minister, the chief executive officer should determine that as an immediate and interim arrangement, subject to review of duties arising out of organisational changes or otherwise, each transferred officer should continue to perform for the health board (and where appropriate, other health boards under an arrangement as provided for in Section 26.2 of the Act), the duties, whether they were expressly defined or not, of his office under a local authority immediately prior to his transfer (including, where appropriate, duties relating to the powers and functions of a local authority as provided for in Section 25 of the Act).

(b) Where a transferred officer was performing, immediately prior to his transfer, either additional duties or the duties of another office in place of the duties of his substantive post which were assigned to him by a local authority on a temporary basis, the reference in sub-paragraph (a) above to the "duties of his office under a local authority" shall be taken to mean his duties prior to the temporary assignment, subject to the continuation of the latter for the period provided for.

Performance of Duties by Deputy

12. (a) Where the chief executive officer gives his consent to any arrangement by a district medical officer, a medical officer of a district hospital or of a fever hospital or of a county home, to perform his duties by a deputy he should limit the periods of

the arrangement to two periods of two days each in any month and an additional half day weekly and no payment should be made by the health board to the deputy.

(b) Apart from the arrangements by the officers mentioned in sub-paragraph (a) the chief executive officer should not give his consent to any arrangement by an officer to perform his duties by a deputy nominated by the officer without the prior approval of the Minister to that arrangement.

Remuneration

13. (a) The chief executive officer may assign remuneration according to their grades to officers and servants at the rates and on the conditions applicable to the respective grades under local authorities immediately prior to the transfer of staff to the service of health boards. The chief executive may also grant allowances to officers and servants in the same circumstances, at the rates and on the conditions which obtained under local authorities prior to the transfer of staff, but only in so far as such allowances were approved by the Minister, not for named officers, but for general application or for application to members in general of a particular grade e.g. allowances payable for acting as a substitute for an officer in a higher grade, allowances payable for possession of special qualifications or for special duties, including 'on call' or 'stand by' allowances. Transferred staff to whom allowances were payable immediately prior to the transfer on a personal basis may continue to be paid such allowances for the period for which and on the conditions on which they were granted.

(b) Any variation in the rates of remuneration or allowances referred to at sub-paragraph (a), payable to an officer or servant or to officers or servants of a specified class, description or grade, and any new grant of an allowance to a named officer or any renewal of a grant to a named officer for a further period shall be subject to the approval of the Minister.

(c) The chief executive officer may pay additional remuneration to officers in appropriate cases in accordance with the provisions of Article 5 of the Local Offices (Irish Language) Regulations, 1966 as if the health board were a local authority.

Starting Pay on Promotion

14. The chief executive officer shall apply the same procedures for dealing with the remuneration of officers on promotion to other offices as applied under local authorities immediately prior to the transfer of staff to the service of health boards.

The following are the provisions:

(i) Where the same salary scale applies to the officer's existing office and the office to which he is being newly appointed, he shall remain on the same point of the scale and may retain his existing incremental date.

(ii) Where the minimum of the new salary scale is greater than existing pay by an amount greater than one increment on the new scale, the officer shall enter the new scale at the minimum—the date of promotion to be the new incremental date.

(iii) Where the minimum of the new salary scale is greater than existing pay by an amount equal to one increment on the new scale, the officer shall enter the new scale at the minimum—he may retain his existing incremental date if any.

(iv) Where the minimum of the new salary scale is greater than existing pay by an amount less than one increment on the new scale, the officer may enter the new scale at the minimum plus one increment—the date of promotion shall be the new incremental date.

(v) Subject to sub-paragraph (i) above, where the minimum of the new salary scale is equal to existing pay, the officer may enter the new scale at the minimum plus one increment—he may retain his existing incremental date, if any.

(vi) Subject to sub-paragraph (i) above, where the minimum of the new salary scale is less than existing pay, the officer may enter the new scale at the point nearest but not below existing pay plus one increment, and

(a) where the point of entry on the new scale is equal to existing pay, he may retain his existing incremental date, if any,

(b) in any other case, the date of promotion shall be the new incremental date.

(vii) Where an officer to whom sub-paragraph (ii) (in cases only where the minimum of the new scale exceeds existing pay by an amount less than two increments on the new scale), (iii), (iv),

(v) or (vi) above applies, has been on a fixed salary or on the maximum of his existing salary scale for at least 3 years at the date of his promotion or new appointment, he may enter the new scale in accordance with the appropriate provision and with a further additional increment, but in that case, the date of promotion or new appointment will be the officer's new incremental date.

(viii) Where after a person has been promoted, and his salary has been determined in accordance with sub-paragraphs (i) to (vii) above, the salary or salary scale applicable to either the officer's former office or his new office, or both, is revised with effect from a date which is earlier than the date of the promotion, the commencing salary shall, subject to sub-paragraphs (ix) and (x) below, be re-determined in accordance with these rules and by reference to the revised salaries or salary scales.

(ix) Where, in a case to which sub-paragraph (viii) applies, the salaries or salary scales of both the officer's former office and his new office are revised with effect from different dates not more than 6 months apart, but only one of the revisions is made effective from a date which is earlier than the date of the promotion or new appointment, the commencing salary shall, subject to sub-paragraph (x), be re-determined as if both revisions had been effective on the date of promotion.

(x) Nothing in sub-paragraphs (i) to (ix) shall be applied so as to enable an officer to have a salary in excess of the maximum salary for the office to which he is promoted or newly appointed.

Travelling expenses and subsistence allowances
15. (a) The chief executive officer shall pay travelling expenses to an officer in respect of every journey necessarily made on official business other than journeys made by a District Medical Officer or a Midwife in connection with his or her attendance on a patient or at a dispensary. The travelling expenses payable shall include
    (i) all reasonable expenses of conveyance properly and necessarily incurred and
    (ii) subsistence allowances where the conditions of subparagraph (d) are met.
(b) No travelling expenses shall be paid in respect of journeys

between an officer's home and his official headquarters i.e. the premises at which he normally performs his duties or such other premises as the chief executive officer may direct in cases of doubt. The chief executive officer may direct in this connection that an officer's home shall be regarded as his official headquarters.

(c) Payment of conveyance expenses where the officer is authorised to use his own car or cycle shall be at the following mileage rates:

Scale A Motor Mileage Rates effective from 1 January 1978

Official mileage in a Mileage year	Inclusive rate per mile		
	Under 10 hp	10 hp and under 12 hp	12 hp and over
Miles	p	p	p
Up to 2000	16.6	19.2	22.0
2001 to 4000	18.2	21.2	24.3
4001 to 6000	9.9	11.0	13.0
6001 to 8000	9.0	10.1	12.2
8001 to 12000	8.3	9.3	10.7
12001 and upwards	7.3	8.2	9.2

(d) The following are the conditions for the payment of subsistence allowances:

(i) where the journey obliges an officer to spend a night away from home a "night allowance" may be paid for each such night. For a continuous period in one place night allowance shall be paid at *normal* rate for the first seven nights, at *reduced* rate for the next 21 nights and at *detention* rate thereafter, as set out in sub-paragraph (f).

(ii) where the journey obliges an officer to remain away from his home for a continuous period of not less than ten hours during the day time, a day allowance may be paid. A reduced day allowance may be paid for five hours but less than ten hours absence.

(e) A day allowance may not be paid in addition to night allowance unless the period of absence is five or ten hours, as the case may be, in excess of a full twenty-four hours absence for each night allowance paid.

(f) The following are the rates at which subsistence allowance (normal, reduced and detention) and day allowances may be paid:

Standard rates of Subsistence

Where the gross annual salary of an officer rises to a figure	Night Allowance			Day Allowance	
	Normal Rate	Reduced Rate	Detention Rate	10 hours or more	5 hours but less than 10 hours
	£	£	£	£	£
Exceeding £7,216 (Class A)	13.21	12.18	6.61	4.40	2.10
Exceeding £4,810 but not exceeding £7,216 (Class B)	11.87	10.16	5.94	3.96	1.79
Not exceeding £4,810 (Class C)	9.94	8.21	4.97	3.31	1.72

(g) The reference in sub-paragraph (a) to journeys on official business includes journeys undertaken in connection with attendance at courses, conferences, seminars, etc., in Ireland recognised and approved by the Minister for Health which the chief executive officer has directed the officer to attend or granted him special leave with pay in order that he may attend.

(h) Where the duties of an officer involve a number of short journeys daily, the chief executive officer may, in lieu of paying travelling expenses, pay a fixed travelling allowance of such amount as in his opinion would not exceed the amount payable in travelling expenses if the latter were payable. Each such travelling allowance shall be fixed for a period not exceeding one year, renewable on review at the end of such period. Where an officer transferred from a local authority to a health board on 1 April 1971 is already in receipt of a fixed travelling allowance he may opt to retain such allowance rather than be paid travelling expenses in accordance with the foregoing paragraphs and shall be entitled to retain such fixed allowance as long as he continues to hold the office in which he has been transferred to the health board.

Application to the Minister by Aggrieved Officers
16. (a) Any officer of a health board who is aggrieved by a decision of his chief executive officer in relation to his terms and conditions of employment, duties, remuneration or allowances, may apply to the Minister to issue a direction to the chief executive officer in relation to such decision and the Minister may issue such direction as he considers appropriate to the chief executive officer in relation to such decision.
(b) An officer who wishes to apply to the Minister to issue a direction to the chief executive officer under Section 14(6) of the Health Act, 1970 shall proceed as follows:
(i) He shall prepare a statement in writing setting out the decision of the chief executive officer by which he is aggrieved and the grounds on which he is so aggrieved;
(ii) he shall send the said statement by registered post to the Minister together with a signed declaration that the facts contained in the said statement are true;
(iii) before sending the said statement to the Minister, he shall give or send by post written notice of the application to the chief executive officer together with a copy of the said statement.

Section 15

Appointments to which the Local Authorities (Officers and Employees) Acts, 1926 and 1940 will apply
17. The Minister has determined, with the consent of the Local Appointments Commissioners, under Section 15(1) of the Health Act, 1970 that the Local Authorities (Officers and Employees) Acts, 1926 and 1940 apply, without any modifications to:
(a) Permanent appointments under a health board corresponding to appointments to the offices under a local authority referred to at Section 2(1)(b) of the Local Authorities (Officers and Employees) Act, 1926, as amended.

Notwithstanding this, the Acts will not apply to any grade of social worker.

(b) Permanent appointments of health inspectors and promotional grades of health inspector.

(c) Permanent appointments of chief nursing officers, matrons, deputy matrons, assistant matrons, head nurses, deputy head nurses in all hospitals and institutions other than

(i) county homes and institutions providing accommodation for similar classes of persons, district hospitals and fever hospitals of less than 100 beds and

(ii) hospitals, other than those mentioned at sub-paragraph (i), in which a religious order is associated with the administration of the hospital.

(d) Permanent appointments of matrons and assistant matrons in hospitals referred to at sub-paragraph (c)(ii), if (i) the appointment is in replacement of an officer who was appointed on the recommendation of the Local Appointments Commissioners or (ii), in any other case, if the appointment is not the appointment of a member of the religious order associated with the administration of the hospital in replacement of another member of that order who had been appointed without advertisement or competition.

(e) Permanent appointments of assistant chief nursing officers in mental hospitals other than an initial appointment following the creation of an office to which a serving permanent officer of the health board is appointed with the Minister's consent.

(f) Permanent appointments of superintendent public health nurses and assistant superintendent public health nurses.

(g) Permanent appointments of director of nursing and assistant director of nursing in centres for the mentally handicapped.

Section 18

Qualifications Generally
18. (a) Except for the appointment of a registered medical practitioner in an additional temporary appointment of the type referred to at paragraph 2(b) no person shall be appointed as an officer who does not possess the qualifications approved of or directed by the Minister for the appointment, subject to

sub-paragraph (b).

(b) Where the chief executive officer experiences difficulty in obtaining suitable persons possessing all the qualifications approved or directed by the Minister for appointments in a particular grade, he may make appointments on a temporary basis without reference to such qualifications insofar as they relate to age or marital status.

Qualifications for Appointment as an Officer

19. (a) The qualifications for appointment as an officer in an existing grade in which officers were transferred from the service of local authorities shall be the qualifications which applied to offices in that grade under local authorities immediately prior to the transfer. Where such qualifications contain an upper age limit and concede an exemption to existing pensionable officers such concessions may be applied to existing pensionable officers of both health boards and local authorities in the State.

(b) Where an appointment as an officer has to be made and no qualifications are applicable to such appointment in accordance with sub-paragraph (a) above, the qualifications proposed by the chief executive officer for the appointment shall be referred to the Minister for approval together with particulars of the nature and extent of the duties for which the appointment is required and other relevant information in regard to the appointment, and the qualifications for the appointment shall be as approved of or directed by the Minister.

(c) The provisions of sub-paragraphs (a) and (b) which relate to appointment of officers, need not be applied to future appointments in grades in which officers have been transferred from the service of local authorities and which had been re-classified under health authorities as grades in which further appointments of officers need not be made. The officers transferred in these grades were appointed prior to the re-classification and should continue as officers. Their replacements and any additional appointments in the grades concerned should not be made as appointments of officers.

Qualifications for continuing as an Officer

20. (a) Where the qualifications for appointment as an officer

referred to in sub-paragraphs 19(a) and (b) include in any case a requirement that the person to be appointed be registered or entitled to be registered in (i) the Register of Medical Practitioners for Ireland, (ii) the Register of Dentists for Ireland, or (iii) the Register of Nurses maintained by An Bord Altranais, the officer appointed in each case must be so registered while continuing as an officer.

(b) A transferred officer who as the holder of an office under a local authority immediately prior to his transfer was required to be registered in the Register of Medical Practitioners for Ireland, or in the Register of Dentists for Ireland, or in the Register of Nurses maintained by An Bord Altranais, must be so registered while continuing as an officer.

(c) Every person appointed to an office in the psychiatric service of a health board as (i) trainee psychiatric nurse or (ii) general trained nurse or (iii) tutor, must be registered in the Psychiatric Nurses Division of the Register of Nurses kept by An Bord Altranais before the expiration of a period of four years after his appointment in the case of (i) and before the expiration of three years after his appointment in the case of (ii) or (iii) as a condition of his continuing as an officer after the termination of such period.

(d) A transferred officer who as the holder of an office of (i) trainee psychiatric nurse, or (ii) general trained nurse in a district mental hospital, or (iii) tutor in a district mental hospital immediately prior to his transfer was required to be registered in the Psychiatric Nurses Division of the Register of Nurses kept by An Bord Altranais within a period of four years in the case of office (i) and three years in the case of office (ii) and office (iii) after his appointment to such office or within such extended period as the Minister may have authorised specially in his case, must comply with such registration requirement within such period or extended period as a condition of his continuing as an officer after the termination of such period or extended period.

(e) A transferred officer who as the holder of an office of assistant medical officer in a district mental hospital immediately prior to his transfer was obliged to acquire a recognised degree or diploma in mental disease or psychological medicine within a period of three years after his appointment to such office or within such extended period as the Minister may have authorised specially in his case, must comply with this requirement within such period or extended period as a condition of his continuing as an officer after the termination of such period or such extended period.

Section 19

Age Limits

21. The Minister has made an order fixing an age higher than 65 years for the purposes of Section 19 of the Health Act, 1970 in respect of each

(a) permanent District Medical Officer;

(b) permanent officer who is transferred to the service of a health board on 1 April 1971 and who immediately before such transfer was the holder of an amalgamated office where such office resulted from the amalgamation of an office of District Medical Officer of a Dispensary District and another office.

(c) permanent officer who if he continues to hold office until he reaches a particular age higher than 65 will then and only then by law be entitled to or be capable of being granted a superannuation allowance on his resigning or otherwise ceasing to hold office, and

(d) permanent officer who is not by law entitled to or capable of being granted a superannuation allowance on his resigning or otherwise ceasing to hold office.

Section 22

Suspensions of Officers and Servants

22. Suspensions of officers and servants will be carried out in accordance with the procedure set out in Section 22 of the Health Act, 1970. Chief Executive Officers are requested to be especially careful to adhere to that procedure.

Sections 23 and 24

Removal of Officers and Servants

23. Removals of officers and servants will be carried out in accordance with Sections 23 and 24 of the Health Act, 1970, and the regulations made under these sections.

Addendum

Circumstances	Conditions
A. All Officers When appointed by a Minister of State to be a member of any Commission, Committee or Statutory Board or a Director of a Company.	Special leave with pay to enable him to attend meetings of the body in question.
When invited by the Local Appointments Commission, Civil Service Commission, a government department, a health board or a local authority, to act on a selection board.	Special leave with pay to enable him to serve on the Board.
For annual training with the Defence Forces/Reserves.	One week with pay; excess over one week, without pay.
Serious illness or death of a near relative.	Up to three days with pay.
When a candidate for a post advertised by the Local Appointments Commission, the Civil Service Commission, a government department, a health board or a local authority.	A maximum of six days with pay in any one year, to enable him to appear before Selection Boards.
For sitting examinations which in the opinion of the chief executive officer are relevant to the work on which the officer is engaged.	The leave necessary for the examination only, with pay.
For attendance at Courses, Conferences, etc., in Ireland recognised and approved by the Minister for Health and of which the chief executive officer is satisfied that they are relevant to the work on which the officer is engaged.	Leave with pay.

For World Health Organisation or Council of Europe Fellowships.

Leave with pay.

B. Medical, Dental and Nursing Officers
For examinations for higher degrees or diplomas.

Fourteen days with pay for study prior to the examination.

To attend clinical meetings of societies appropriate to their specialties.

Not more than seven days in any one year, with pay.

APPENDIX C

Estimated Non-Capital Expenditure, 1977, allocated by Programmes and Services

Programme and Service		Amount (£ Million)
Community Protection Programme		
1.1 Prevention of infectious diseases		2.120
1.2 Child health examinations		3.950
1.3 Food hygiene and standards		0.640
1.4 Drugs Advisory Board		0.120
1.5 Health Education		0.400
1.6 Other preventive services		0.370
	Total	7.600
	Less Income	0.130
	Net Total	7.470
Community Health Services Programme		
2.1 General Practitioner services (including prescribed drugs)		35.200
2.2 Subsidies for drugs purchases by patients ineligible under 2.1		1.650
2.3 Refund of cost of drugs for long-term illnesses (including hardship cases)		1.600
2.4 Home nursing services		2.520
2.5 Domiciliary maternity service		1.010
2.6 Dental Services		3.520
2.7 Ophthalmic services		0.720
2.8 Aural services		0.260
	Total	46.480
	Less Income	1.200
	Net Total	45.280

Programme and Service		Amount ($£$ million)

Community Welfare Programme

3.1	Cash payments to disabled persons	16.711
3.2	Cash payments to persons with certain infectious diseases	0.460
3.3	Maternity cash grants	0.150
3.4	Allowances for 'constant care' of disabled children	1.400
3.5	Cash payments to blind persons	0.385
3.6	Home help services	1.565
3.7	Meals-on-wheels service	0.750
3.8	Grants to voluntary welfare agencies	2.220
3.9	Supply of free milk	0.600
3.10	Boarding-out of children	0.400
3.11	Payments for children in 'approved schools'	1.495
3.12	Welfare homes for the aged	1.423

Total	27.559
Less Income	0.459
Net Total	27.100

Occupational Rehabilitation

4.1	Rehabilitation service	

Total	1.540
Less Income	0.020
Net Total	1.520

Psychiatric Programme

5.1	Service for diagnosis, care and prevention of psychiatric ailments	

Total	46.500
Less Income	4.150
Net Total	42.350

Programme and Service		Amount (£ million)
Mental Handicap Programme		
6.1 Care in special homes		13.200
6.2 Care in psychiatric hospitals		8.800
6.3 Care in day centres		0.840
	Total	22.840
	Less Income	1.013
	Net Total	21.827
Physical Handicap Programme		
7.1 Assessment and care of blind		0.515
7.2 Assessment and care of deaf		0.440
7.3 Assessment and care of persons otherwise handicapped		4.770
	Total	5.725
	Less Income	0.120
	Net Total	5.605
General Hospitals Programme		
8.1 Services in regional hospitals (excluding voluntary)		33.950
8.2 Services in public voluntary hospitals		72.250
8.3 Services in health board county hospitals		29.900
8.4 Services in private voluntary hospitals		4.620
8.5 Services in district hospitals		7.890
8.6 Services in health board long-stay hospitals		19.600
8.7 Services in voluntary long-stay hospitals		1.025
8.8 Ambulance services		3.800
	Total	173.035
	Less Income	17.500
	Net Total	155.535

Programme and Service		Amount ($£$ million)
General Support Programme		
9.1 Central Administration		2.680
9.2 Local Administration		7.400
9.3 Research		0.700
9.4 Superannuation		5.200
9.5 Interest and other financial arrangements		8.300
	Total	24.280
	Less Income	2.500
	Net Total	21.780
Total for all programmes		355.559
Less Income		27.092
Net Total		328.467

Full Eligibility

I. Standard Guidelines for Full Eligibility (1 January 1979)

Income limits

Single person living alone:	weekly income of £28 or less
Single person living with family	weekly income of £24 or less
Married couple:	weekly income of £40.50 or less

Allowances added to limits

For each child under sixteen years:	£4
For each other dependant:	£5.50
For weekly outgoings on house: excess over reasonable expenses necessarily incurred in travel to work:	£4
Other allowance	Reasonable expenses necessarily incurred in travelling to work

II. Distribution of persons with full eligibility on a health board and county basis:

	Number of Persons (including dependants) covered by Medical Cards on 31 March 1978		Number of Persons (including dependants) covered by Medical Cards on 31 March 1978
Eastern		*Midland*	
Dublin	206,560	Longford	16,034
Wicklow	24,330	Westmeath	25,845
Kildare	28,810	Offaly	28,174
		Laois	22,152
TOTAL	259,700	TOTAL	92,205
Mid Western		*North Eastern*	
Clare	31,176	Cavan	30,242
Limerick	62,567	Louth	33,155
Tipperary (NR)	20,886	Meath	33,441
		Monaghan	25,269
TOTAL	114,629	TOTAL	122,107
North Western		*South Eastern*	
Donegal	77,372	Carlow	17,298
Leitrim	17,267	Kilkenny	30,423
Sligo	27,096	Tipperary (SR)	33,422
		Waterford	34,104
		Wexford	41,878
TOTAL	121,735	TOTAL	157,125
Southern		*Western*	
Cork	121,184	Galway	88,630
Kerry	54,338	Mayo	71,481
		Roscommon	31,280
TOTAL	175,522	TOTAL	191,391
		GRAND TOTAL	1,234,414

III. Classification of Persons (including dependants) with Full
Eligibility on 31 March, 1978.

	Numbers	Percentage
Farmers	122,948	9.96
Other Self-employed	19,998	1.62
Farm Labourers	36,786	2.98
Other Wage Earners	270,213	21.89
Students	98,012	7.94
Unemployed	275,027	22.28
Welfare recipients	381,187	30.88
Other	30,243	2.45
Total	1,234,414	100.00

APPENDIX E

Summary of Provisions on Infectious Diseases

[NOTE: *The regulations referred to below are due to be replaced by more modern versions.*]

Definition of Infectious Diseases

The Minister for Health has power 'by regulation to specify the diseases which are infectious diseases' and to define a disease in such regulations 'in any manner which he considers suitable including, in particular, by reference to any stage of the disease or by reference to any class of sufferers from the disease'.[1] Diseases are specified and defined in the exercise of this power merely for the purpose of stating the diseases to which the service applies; the omission of a disease from the list does not mean that the Minister is attempting to influence medical opinion as to its nature. In fact, where convenience in the operation of the service demands, diseases are periodically added to and taken from the list. When smallpox threatened in 1949 and 1952, chicken-pox was temporarily added to the list and acute lymphocytic meningitis was similarly included when poliomyelitis was prevalent in the Autumn of 1956.[2] The complete list of the specified infectious diseases is as follows:[3]

acute anterior poliomyelitis.
acute lymphocytic meningitis.
anthrax.
brucellosis.
cerebro-spinal fever.
cholera.
diphtheria.
dysentery.
encephalitis lethargica.
epidemic diarrhoea and enteritis (under two years).
erysipelas.
gonorrhoea.
haemorrhagic jaundice (Weil's disease).
impetigo contagiosa.
infectious hepatitis.

[1]Section 29 of the Health Act, 1947.
[2]These were added by the Infectious Diseases (Temporary Provisions) Regulations 1949, 1952 and 1956. The first two of these sets of regulations were revoked after being a few months in operation.
[3]See the Second Schedule to the Infectious Diseases Regulations, 1948.

infective mononucleosis.

influenza.

influenzal pneumonia.

lassa fever.[4]

malaria.

measles.

ophthalmia neonatorum.

paratyphoid A.

paratyphoid B.

pemphigus neonatorum.

plague.

primary pneumonia.

psittacosis.

puerperal pyrexia.

puerperal sepsis.

rabies.[4]

rubella.

salmonella infection.[5]

scabies.

scarlet fever.

smallpox.

soft chancre.

streptococcal sore-throat.

syphilis.

tinea capitis.

tuberculosis.

trachoma.

typhoid.

typhus.

whooping cough.

yellow fever.

The complete control service and its ancillary benefits (such as maintenance allowances) do not extend to all of these diseases. Neither are they all notifiable. The exceptions will be mentioned later.

Notification[6]

Diseases other than tuberculosis and venereal disease
All the diseases on the above list except impetigo contagiosa, influenza, primary pneumonia and streptococcal sore-throat[7] are notifiable. Scabies is notifiable only when it occurs in an urban area. The system of notification for tuberculosis and the venereal diseases is somewhat different from that for the other infectious diseases. It is as well to deal with the latter diseases first.

A medical practitioner must notify the appropriate medical officer,[8] as soon as he becomes aware or suspects that a person on whom he is in professional attendance (otherwise than as a

[4] These diseases were added by article 2 of the Infectious Diseases (Amendment) Regulations, 1976.

[5] This disease was added by article 4 of the Infectious Diseases (Amendment) Regulations, 1948.

[6] The succeeding paragraphs summarise Part V of the Infectious Diseases Regulations, 1948, as amended by article 2 of the Infectious Diseases (Amendment) Regulations, 1949.

[7] This disease was excluded by the Infectious Diseases (Amendment) Regulations, 1951.

[8] In accordance with article 3 of the Health Act, 1970 (Adaptation) Regulations, 1971, this is the medical officer of the health board carrying out duties formerly performed by a county medical officer.

medical officer of an infectious disease institution) is suffering from or is a carrier of one of these other infectious diseases. The notification is made on a prescribed form (supplies of which are made available by the health boards) and is posted in a sealed envelope to the medical officer. Where there is an occurrence of one of the more virulent diseases (poliomyelitis, cerebro-spinal fever, cholera, plague, psittacosis, puerperal sepsis, smallpox, typhus or yellow fever) or where a serious out-break of any disease is suspected the medical practitioner must also give an immediate preliminary notification by telephone or telegram to the medical officer. Where a doctor has notified his suspicion that a case is one of an infectious disease, he must (unless the patient has gone into an infectious disease hospital) tell the medical officer when his suspicion is confirmed or cancelled. Where a patient is sent to hospital, the terms of the notification to the medical officer must be communicated to the medical officer of the hospital. The medical officer of an infec-tious disease hospital need not normally notify cases admitted for treatment unless the patient's disease was first definitely diagnosed in the hospital, or was contracted in the hospital.

It is not, of course, practicable to get notification of all the cases of infectious diseases as some may not receive medical attention at all. There is a provision in the regulations, however, which requires the person in charge of a place such as a school, hotel, factory or office to tell the medical officer of any suspected case of infectious disease in the establishment which is not being attended by a medical practitioner.

Notification of tuberculosis

Tuberculosis in any of its forms is a notifiable disease. Only confirmed cases need be notified, however, and medical officers of sanatoria or hospitals treating tuberculosis cases need not notify them.

Suspected cases of tuberculosis may be 'intimated' to the medical officer. This intimation is, in fact, a request to have a suspected case examined under the Tuberculosis Service. Where such an examination is arranged, the patient's doctor gets a confidential report on it.

Notification of venereal disease

The venereal diseases are notifiable but the special forms used do not divulge the patient's name or address to the medical officer. He becomes aware only that a case exists. Three months after such a notification is made, the notifying doctor must send in a report showing whether the patient has been treated or not. The aim of this scheme of notification is to get more accurate information on the incidence of venereal diseases and the willingness of those suffering from them to take treatment.

Fees for notification

A fee is payable by the health board to the notifying doctor for each notification of a case which is confirmed as infectious. The fee is 25p for each notification of venereal disease and $12\frac{1}{2}$p for other notifications. The cost of telegrams and telephone calls is also refunded by the health board.

Returns of infectious diseases

Each medical officer must send to the Minister for Health, by Monday or, at the latest, Tuesday morning, each week a return of the cases of infectious diseases notified to him. He must also furnish detailed reports on cases of some diseases specified by the Minister.

Diagnosis and Treatment

Health boards are required 'to make arrangements for the diagnosis and treatment of infectious disease in persons in their district'. No charge can be made for any service given under these arrangements except where superior services (such as maintenance in a private or semi-private ward) are provided on request.[9]

Treatment is generally given in the health boards' hospitals, but some other hospitals are also used. Free treatment outside hospital at general practitioner level is not part of the service, but the health board may provide nurses for domiciliary cases. Charges may be made for the services of such nurses.[10]

[9]See article 12 of the Infectious Diseases Regulations, 1948.
[10]See section 42 of the Health Act, 1947.

Prevention of the Spread of Infection[11]

A number of penal obligations to take precautions against the spread of infection are imposed by the Health Act, 1947, and the Infectious Diseases Regulations. A person who 'knows that he is a probable source of infection with an infectious disease' must, in addition to taking the specific precautions mentioned below, 'take every other reasonable precaution to prevent his infecting others with such disease by his presence or conduct or by means of any article with which he has been in contact'. Similar precautions must be taken as respects a person in one's care who is a probable source of infection. The penalty prescribed is a fine of up to £50.

Furthermore, where a civil action arises out of one person being infected through another not taking the precautions prescribed, it is provided that the court will assume that the latter was the cause of the infection being spread unless he can prove that the circumstances were such that it was unlikely that his failure to take precautions led to the other person getting the disease.

A number of specific obligations—no longer of much practical importance—are imposed by the Act where a dwelling or room is being sold, let or occupied within three months of the occurrence in it of a case of tuberculosis or typhus.[12]

A parent who 'knows that his child is suffering from or is a probable source of infection with an infectious disease' may not allow him to attend school or college except with the permission of the local medical officer and in accordance with any conditions he may impose.

There are restrictions on the use of public conveyances (these include taxis and hackney cars) by a person suffering from poliomyelitis, cerebro-spinal fever, diphtheria, measles, typhoid or paratyphoid, scarlet fever, smallpox or typhus. A patient with any of these diseases may not 'enter a public conveyance used for the conveyance of passengers at separate fares' (for example, a train or bus) and he may not use a taxi or hackney un-

[11]The following paragraphs summarise section 30, sections 33 to 37 and section 43 of the Health Act, 1947, articles 13 to 21 of the Infectious Diseases Regulations, 1948, article 3 of the Infectious Diseases (Amendment) Regulations, 1948 and the Infectious Diseases (Amendment) Regulations, 1952.
[12]The application of sections 33 to 36 of the 1947 Act (which impose these obligations) is limited to these diseases by article 8 of the Infectious Diseases Regulations, 1948.

less the person in charge of it knows about the disease and agrees to take the patient as a passenger. Where he does so, the person in charge can insist on prior payment of a sum sufficient to meet the expense of disinfection. Where the owner of a public conveyance learns that a person suffering from one of the diseases mentioned has been carried in it, he must immediately take it out of service, tell the medical officer and have the conveyance disinfected to the latter's satisfaction before putting it to use again.

Powers of medical officers

The medical officers of the health boards have wide powers to supplement these precautions where cases of infection have occurred or are suspected. The medical officer is obliged to 'make such enquiries and take such steps as are necessary or desirable for investigating the nature and source of the infection, for preventing the spread of infection and for removing conditions favourable to infection'. This he may do himself or through the agency of his subordinate officers.

Having regard to the circumstances of the case and the nature of the disease, the medical officer may require a person to stay in his home (and, perhaps, isolate himself there), to remain away from any specified place or to discontinue certain occupations. He may require the cleansing, disinfection or disinfestation of persons, buildings, structures, vehicles, vessels, aircraft or articles.

Measures for the destruction of animals or insects may also be imposed. The medical officer, in the course of his investigations, may arrange for the compulsory medical examination of any person (where possible after due notice to him and to suit his convenience). The person concerned or the parent of a child must facilitate such an examination and is required to permit the taking of blood or other specimens for examinations or tests.

The medical officer may require the destruction or suitable disposal of substances or articles which are infected, infested or dirty or which have been imported from a country where there has been a serious outbreak of infectious disease and are likely to harbour infection. The health board is obliged to provide facilities for cleansing, disinfection and disinfestation.

Isolation of infective persons

If the medical officer is satisfied that the isolation of a person who is a probable source of infection with poliomyelitis, cholera, diphtheria, gonorrhoea, syphilis, smallpox, tuberculosis, typhoid, paratyphoid or typhus[13] is necessary and that the person cannot be effectively isolated at home, he may make an order directing the person's detention and isolation in some other place. Such an order is not effective, however, unless it is signed by another medical practitioner as well as the officer.[14]

Where a detention order has been made, the person concerned may be taken to the hospital or other place named in it and kept there until the medical officer gives a certificate that he is no longer a probable source of infection. A detained person (or, where he is a child, his parent) may, however, appeal to the Minister for Health against the detention and the latter may direct his release.[15]

Immunisation and Vaccination[16]

Health boards may purchase and keep supplies of any diagnostic or immunising agents approved by the Minister and may operate schemes for the administration of these agents to the public. They may also make such agents available to medical practitioners 'on such reasonable terms as the health authority may determine'.

The Health Act, 1947, repealed the Vaccination Acts under which vaccination against smallpox had been compulsory on all infants. Now the law on vaccination[17] requires that the medical officer sends a notice to the parent of each infant requesting the parent to submit him for vaccination. The parent commits an offence in not bringing the child for vaccination unless he sends in, before the time set, a written objection to vaccination, a statement that the child's health is such that he thinks it would

[13] Article 9 of the Infectious Diseases Regulations, 1948 limits the application of section 38 of the 1947 Act to these diseases.

[14] See section 35 of the Health Act, 1953.

[15] This is but a brief synopsis of the procedure for compulsory detention. Any medical officer contemplating the use of his powers under the section would need to study in detail the procedure, which is set out at length in section 38 of the Health Act, 1947 (as amended by section 35 of the 1953 Act). The powers, in fact, have been used very little up to the present.

[16] The law on immunisation and vaccination is contained principally in Part IV of the Infectious Diseases Regulations, 1948. This is based on sections 31 and 32 of the Health Act, 1947.

[17] Article 24 of the Infectious Diseases Regulations, 1948.

not be proper to vaccinate him or a medical certificate, that certificate being to the effect that the child has been vaccinated within three years or that two attempted vaccinations have been unsuccessful. The object of this change in the law was to replace the absolute compulsion of the Vaccination Acts with a scheme under which parents' objections would be respected, but the onus of making an objection was placed on the parent. If the child is at the clinic at the time mentioned in the notice and if an objection or medical certificate has not been submitted, the parent is 'deemed to have submitted him for vaccination'. In fact, these provisions on vaccination against smallpox did not operate any better than did the old Vaccination Acts, which had never been fully observed in Ireland.

Should it seem necessary for the purpose of preventing the spread of smallpox, the Minister may make an order which would make it an offence for a parent to withhold a child from vaccination except on a medical certificate. Regulations can also make vaccination of airport and seaport workers compulsory at any time without right of exemption.[18]

At the option of the medical officer a similar 'semi-compulsory scheme' could be operated for immunisation against diphtheria. In practice, however, this is not done. Diphtheria immunisation schemes, like those for BCG, poliomyelitis and rubella vaccination, are operated on a voluntary basis.

International Health Regulations

Under the International Health Regulations[19] which were adopted by the World Health Organisation in 1951, each member State of the Organisation is obliged to take steps to keep the Organisation informed of the occurrence of outbreaks of plague, cholera, smallpox or yellow fever and to take steps to prevent these diseases from spreading to other countries. The Regulations oblige the health administrations to provide at ports and airports the facilities necessary for taking the prescribed measures to prevent the diseases referred to from spreading. The maximum steps which any member State of the World Health Organisation may take with the aim of

[18]See section 34 of the Health Act, 1953.
[19]These Regulations, like other WHO publications, may be bought from the Government Publications Sale Office, G.P.O. Arcade, Dublin.

protecting its territory against the diseases are delimited. Sanitary measures must be completed without unnecessary delay to traffic and must be carried out so as not to cause undue discomfort to any person, or injury to health, and not to damage the structure of ships or aircraft. What may be done by the local health authorities in respect of departing and arriving vessels and aircraft is specified in considerable detail, as are the measures which may be taken in respect of each of the diseases covered by the Regulations.

These Regulations have been accepted by most member States of the Organisation. They replace a number of International Sanitary Conventions and Agreements, dating back to 1903. So far as Ireland is concerned, the health regulations governing sea and air traffic, which were made in 1948, and the administrative practices are in conformity with the International Health Regulations.

Infectious Diseases (Shipping) Regulations, 1948

Since it became known or suspected that some diseases could be spread by contact with persons on board ships from foreign ports, steps were taken in each civilised country to watch incoming ships and to take measures to stop the entry of infection. Strict quarantine of the ship and all aboard was originally the only effective safeguard known but, with increasing knowledge as to how the different infectious diseases are spread, less drastic but equally effective measures are imposed. The Infectious Diseases (Shipping) Regulations specify what these measures are in the case of Ireland.

Masters of foreign-going ships are required to give notice (in advance of arrival if possible) of any case of illness on board which has the symptoms of any infectious disease on a list scheduled in the Regulations.[20] Whether or not there is such case on board, the master must display a flag signal indicating either that the ship is healthy or that it is not and he must deliver a declaration of health to the customs and excise officer or health officer who first boards the ship on arrival. No one may, without the permission of the health officer, board or

---

[20]The diseases are—acute anterior poliomyelitis, anthrax, cerebro-spinal fever, cholera, diphtheria, dysentery, malaria, measles, plague, psittacosis, scarlet fever, smallpox, typhoid or paratyphoid, typhus or yellow fever.

leave the ship in port until it has been freed from control under the Regulations.

These requirements do not normally apply to ships trading with an 'excepted area' which includes Great Britain, Northern Ireland, the Isle of Man, the Channel Islands and much of Western Europe,[21] but such ships, in common with foreign-going ships, may be subjected to detention and the passengers and crew to prescribed preventive measures if a case of infection occurs on board.

Rats being carriers of plague, it is very important that ships in international trade should be kept free of them. The Regulations, in conformity with international requirements, thus specify that any arriving ship without a 'deratting certificate' or 'deratting exemption certificate' issued within the previous six (or, in some cases, seven) months must, if necessary, be 'deratted'.

The medical officer for each port also has obligations in respect of outgoing traffic. He may examine any person embarking and prohibit anyone showing symptoms of any of the scheduled diseases from embarking. Depending on the nature of the diseases, other precautions may be taken.

Infectious Diseases (Aircraft) Regulations, 1948
The obligations placed on aircraft commanders and the powers and duties of medical officers at airports are similar to those laid down in the case of shipping. Any aircraft arriving from outside the 'excepted area'[21] must, if required, present a declaration of health and all arriving and departing aircraft are subject to prescribed controls where a case of infectious disease is aboard.

[21]The excepted area at present comprises all the territory of Belgium, Metropolitan France, Greece, Ireland, Italy, Luxembourg, the Netherlands and the United Kingdom (England, Wales, Scotland, Northern Ireland, the Channel Islands and the Isle of Man).

APPENDIX F

Summary of Provisions on Food and Drugs[1]

The Food Hygiene Regulations[2]

The purpose of these regulations is to prohibit and prevent the sale of diseased or contaminated food and to prescribe hygienic precautions for the manufacture, preparation, sale and serving of food. 'Food' in the context of the regulations includes 'every article used for food or drink by man, other than drugs or water' and also includes ingredients of foods, flavouring or colouring matters, preservatives and condiments.[3] The penalty for breaking the Regulations may be a fine of £100, with £10 a day for a continuing offence, or imprisonment for a term up to six months, or both fine and imprisonment.

Sale, etc., of unfit food
There is a general prohibition on the sale of unfit food, in the following terms:—

'No person shall sell or offer or keep for sale:—
(a) any article of food intended for human consumption,

(b) any food animal or

(c) any food material

which is diseased, contaminated or otherwise unfit for human consumption'.[4]
This is supplemented by a provision making it an offence to sell or use in the manufacture or preparation of food any food or

---

[1]The law on these matters is contained in Part V and section 65 of the Health Act, 1947 (as amended by section 38 of the Health Act, 1953), the Sale of Food and Drugs Acts 1875 to 1936, the Poisons (Ireland) Act, 1870, the Poisons and Pharmacy Act, 1908, the Therapeutic Substances Act, 1932, the Dangerous Drugs Act, 1934, the Poisons Act, 1961, section 78 of the Health Act, 1970 and the several sets of regulations made under these Acts.
[2]The Food Hygiene Regulations, 1950 to 1971, were made under section 54 of the Health Act, 1947 and section 55 of that Act, as amended by section 38 of the Health Act, 1953.
[3]See section 53 of the Health Act, 1947.
[4]Article 9 of the 1950 Regulations.

ingredient known to have been exposed to infection with a scheduled infectious disease.[5]

Here it is as well to say that the terminology of the Food Hygiene Regulations is based on a considerable number of interlocking artificial definitions.[6] 'Food animal' and 'food material' are among these definitions. The former means a dead farm animal (which animals are in turn defined as 'cattle, sheep, pigs, goats and poultry as defined in the Agricultural Produce (Fresh Meat) Act, 1930') or any other animal, whether living or dead, intended for food for human consumption. 'Food material' means 'any material or article which is used or intended for use in the preparation or manufacture of food intended for human consumption and which may enter into the composition of food'. These two definitions are cited because this is necessary for the comprehension of the important provisions referred to in the preceding paragraph. There are, however, no less than forty definitions of this nature in the Regulations and it would not be possible to follow the intricacies of all of these in explaining what is contained in the rest of the Regulations.

Seizure of unfit food[7]

An 'authorised officer' (generally a health inspector or veterinary officer) may seize, remove and detain food, food animals or food material which he suspects to be diseased, contaminated or otherwise unfit for human consumption. Where this is done, the article or animal may be destroyed there and then if the owner or person in charge agrees; if he does not, destruction or other disposal is contingent on an order of a District Justice or a Peace Commissioner.

The provisions relating to the sale of unfit food do not, in general, apply to a number of agricultural products such as milk, pigs, where they are controlled under legislation administered by the Department of Agriculture. The power to seize, remove and detain and the prohibition on transactions

---

[5]See article 10 of the 1950 Regulations. The scheduled infectious diseases are: acute anterior poliomyelitis, diphtheria, dysentery, salmonella infection, scarlet fever, streptococcal sore-throat, tuberculosis, typhoid and paratyphoid. See the Second Schedule to the 1950 Regulations.
[6]See article 2 of the 1950 Regulations.
[7]Article 11 of 1950 Regulations.

in food exposed to infection apply, however, to these products in the same way as to other foods.

Importation of Unfit Food[8]

An importer of any food, food animal or food material who discovers that it is diseased, contaminated or otherwise unfit for human consumption, must so inform the local medical officer (or, in the case of cereals, a cereals officer of the Department of Agriculture), do what that officer directs as to where and how it may be stored and, in accordance with the specification of the officer, destroy, re-export, re-condition or otherwise deal with it. Where the medical officer (or the cereals officer) has advance information to the effect that an article of food, food animal or food material is unfit for human consumption, he may make an order prohibiting its importation or, where it has been landed, its removal from the place of importation. There is an appeal to a District Justice or a Peace Commissioner against such an order.

There are special controls on the importation of meat.

The prohibitions and controls on import in the Food Hygiene Regulations do not apply to posted articles or to food in the personal baggage of the importer. Neither do they apply to food, food animals or food material for consumption on a vehicle, ship or aircraft.

Powers of inspection, sampling, etc.[9]

Enforcing officers have wide powers of inspection and those in charge of food or food businesses must facilitate them in their inspections. Samples of food, of materials used in preparing food or of by-products of food manufacture may be taken without payment by the medical officer or other authorised officer and where a sample has been taken, the officer may direct a standstill on movement of the consignment until the result of the test on the sample is known. Persons carrying on food businesses must give the authorised officer all reasonable assistance and information, including information on the origin and destination of their purchases and sales (retail traders however would not be expected to record the names of the purchasers of their goods).

[8]Chapter II of Part II of the 1950 Regulations.
[9]Chapter III of Part II of the 1950 Regulations.

Control of manufacture, retail trade, etc.[10]

With the exception of food processes and transactions controlled by the Department of Agriculture under its own legislation, all manufacture, preparation, handling, serving, selling and transport of food is subject to control under the Regulations. Over twenty different 'shalls' and 'shall-nots' are set out for the proprietors of food premises, ranging from a requirement for the 'walls, ceilings, floors, doors, windows and all parts of the premises' to be 'kept in a proper state of repair and in a clean and hygienic condition' to the exclusion of cats and dogs (except in certain circumstances). Ventilation, lighting, water supply, washing facilities, drainage, sanitary accommodation and refuse disposal are also covered. Machinery must be 'constructed and adjusted so as to prevent the contamination of food or food material by dirt from the mechanism' and chipped or cracked ware may not be used to serve food. Precautions must be taken against the contamination of food 'by foreign matter or unnecessary handling or by rats, mice or insects or otherwise' and unsuitable wrapping materials are barred. As a complement to these and the other specific prohibitions, article 25 of the Regulations concludes by requiring the proprietor of the food premises to 'take every other reasonable precaution to prevent danger to the public health arising from the food business and to prevent the contamination of food in the food premises'.

Stalls and vehicles from which food is sold are expected to comply with similar conditions and those selling food 'otherwise than at a food premises or a food stall' (i.e. those carrying it in a box or basket) are also governed by the Regulations. Vehicles in which food is transported must be properly constructed and kept clean and, in their use, adequate steps must be taken to prevent the contamination of food. Containers in which food is carried must also be properly constructed and cared for and food ready to be eaten (such as bread) must be carried in a covered container.

Each worker in a food business is required to keep himself clean, to keep the equipment he uses in a clean and hygienic condition, to refrain from doing anything to contaminate the food on which he works and generally to take all reasonable

[10]Part III of the 1950 Regulations.

precautions to prevent danger to the public health arising from his work. Visitors to places where food is being prepared must observe like precautions.

A person likely to cause infection with any of the scheduled infectious diseases[11] or who has a boil, septic sore or other skin ailment on the hand or forearm which could contaminate food may not work in a food business except with the permission of the local medical officer. The proprietor must ask anyone who intends to take up employment in a food business whether he is a probable source of infection with a scheduled infectious disease or whether he ever suffered from typhoid or paratyphoid. The person seeking employment must answer this question to the best of his knowledge.

[All these requirements may seem to place those in the food business in constant and continuous danger of prosecution. In fact, however, many of the provisions are such as would be observed in any event by decent and competent manufacturers and dealers. Furthermore, health inspectors endeavour in the first place to educate food traders to observe the Regulations. Prosecution is not resorted to for all violations and, generally speaking, an offender will be brought to court only where there is deliberate and dangerous violation of the code of food hygiene.]

To deal with a case where there is a grave and immediate danger to public health from conditions in a premises or vehicle or at a stall, the Minister has power to make an order directing the immediate cessation of the use of the premises, vehicle or stall for the purposes of a food business. There is an appeal to the District Justice against such an order.

Registration of food premises[12]

Registration of all the premises to which the provisions mentioned under the preceding heading apply is provided for, but the scheme of registration can be applied piecemeal by Minister's order to different areas and different classes of premises.[13] When registration is applied to any type of

[11]See footnote 5.
[12]Part IV of 1950 Regulations as amended.
[13]To date, hotels, holiday camps and restaurants and fishmongers', poulterers', butchers', pork butchers', ice-cream makers', manufacturers' and wholesalers' premises have been registered (see Food Hygiene Regulations, 1950 (Commencement of Part IV) Order, 1951).

premises, there follows a period of a year during which proprietors apply for registration, the health board tells each one if any alterations to the premises are called for and any such alterations can be made. The requirement to be registered becomes effective at the end of the year and before then the health board will have dealt with each application by registering the premises, granting provisional registration for a period up to six months, or refusing registration on stated grounds. At the end of the period for which it is granted, provisional registration can be made no longer provisional, can be withdrawn, or can be extended for one more period.

There is an appeal to the Minister against a decision of the chief executive officer of a health board not to register a premises and, for those who were in business when registration was ordained for the particular class of premises, a further appeal lies to a District Justice. After the expiration of the year of grace, no one can carry on a food business of a type specified in the commencement order in a premises which is not registered. Persons wishing to start any such businesses thereafter should apply for and obtain registration before they commence to operate.

Registration attaches to the premises and not to the proprietor. When a business changes hands, the health board merely alters the name in their register.

Where a registered proprietor of a food premises is convicted of an offence under Part III of the Regulations (which are summarised under the preceding heading), the health board is called upon to see during the following year whether the neglect to comply with this Part of the Regulations continues. If it does, the board may ask the Minister to order the cancellation of the registration. When so asked (or when satisfied from enquiries initiated by himself), the Minister may make an order cancelling or suspending registration. An appeal to annul any such order may be made to the District Justice.

'Occasional' food premises

Premises where a food business is carried on only occasionally[14] are not subject to the full requirements of registration. Special

[14]The definition of 'occasional food premises' (article 2 of 1950 Regulations) is 'a food premises in which a food business is carried on for not more than two months at any time and for not more than four months in any calendar year'.

permits are issued by health boards for each occasional use of a premises.

Hygiene of ice-cream[15]

To supplement the general provisions of the Regulations, there are special requirements in the preparation of ice-cream. 'Heat-treatment' of the mix, or the use of safe ingredients, is prescribed and the temperatures at which the mix be kept before being made into ice-cream are specified.[16] Frequent recordings of temperatures are required in the making and storing of ice-cream and suitable thermometers must be installed for this purpose.

Shellfish[17]

To avoid typhoid being transmitted by oysters, clams, cockles, mussels or similar shellfish or periwinkles taken from areas which might be polluted by sewage, the sale of these shellfish is controlled. Purification of such shellfish by an approved method before sale is required where they have been taken from a 'controlled area'. Persons dealing in shellfish must keep records of where the fish come from and, except for retailers, to whom they are sold.

Sale of Food and Drugs Act

The Sale of Food and Drugs Acts 1875 to 1936[18] were designed to prevent the sale of food or drugs which are injurious to health or 'not of the nature, substance and quality demanded by the purchaser'. Food and drugs inspectors are appointed by

[15]Part V of 1950 Regulations, as amended by the 1971 Regulations.
[16]With heat treatment, the mix may not be kept for more than an hour between 45°F. and 150°F. before being subjected to the treatment (which is the keeping of the temperature at 150°F. or higher for at least thirty minutes or at 160°F. or higher for at least fifteen minutes or, in special cases, such other temperature for such period as may be approved by the Minister) and, after the treatment, it must be brought down to 45°F. or lower within one-and-a-half hours and kept below that temperature. Where the mix is prepared without heat-treatment (i.e. by using the specified safe ingredients), it must be frozen within an hour of being wetted and thereafter kept below 45°F.
[17]Part VI of 1950 Regulations. The controlled areas (which adjoin parts of the coasts of Cork, Galway, Kerry, Louth, Mayo, Sligo, Waterford and Wexford) are specified in the Food Hygiene Regulations, 1950 (Shellfish Controlled Areas) Orders, 1951, 1952, 1971 and 1977.
[18]A complete list of the Acts and the Regulations is given in Appendix J. The basic provisions are in sections 3 to 19 of the Act of 1875.

the health boards. These are mainly health inspectors. Public analysts are employed by the health boards to report on samples taken under the Acts.

A food and drugs inspector (or any other person who wishes to do so at his own expense) may purchase a sample of any food or drug and submit it for analysis. The sample is first divided in three. One part is sent for analysis; another is given to the vendor (who must be told that the sample is to be analysed) and the third part is kept by the inspector for future comparison. The Court, where proceedings are taken under the Act, may order this part of the sample to be sent to the State Chemist, as referee. Proceedings are normally taken by the inspector who took the sample.

Special provisions are included in respect of milk, butter and margarine. Milk is regarded as not being of the 'nature, substance and quality' demanded by the purchaser if it does not contain prescribed percentages of milk-fat and other milk solids.[19] Similar provisions relate to cream, buttermilk and skimmed milk. Butter or margarine may not contain more than 16% of water. Margarine may not contain more than 10% of butter fat and its wrapper must also be conspicuously marked so as to distinguish it from butter.

Food Standards[20]

The Minister for Health, if of opinion that the composition of any food is of special importance to the public health, may, under the Health Act, 1947, prescribe a standard for the chemical composition of that food. The only standard so far laid down in the exercise of this power is that for ice-cream.[21] In addition to the powers conferred on him under the Health Act, 1947, the

---

[19]The percentages are prescribed in the Milk (Percentages of Milk-fat and Milk-solids) (No. 2) Regulations, 1936. The percentages are: for milk 3% milk fat and 8·5% other milk solids; for cream 25% milk fat; for skimmed milk 8·6% milk solids not fat and for buttermilk 6·2% milk solids not fat.

[20]See sections 56, 57 and 63 of the Health Act, 1947 (as amended by section 38 of the 1953 Act).

[21]This standard was fixed by the Food Standards (Ice-cream) Regulations, 1952. It requires at least 5% milk fat, 9% other milk solids and 10% sugar (by weight in each case) in ice-cream.

Minister for Health is also empowered, under the Food Standards Act, 1974, to prescribe standards for food.[22]

Additives and Contaminants in Food

The use of additives in food (preservatives, colouring agents, antioxidants and solvents) and the presence of undesirable substances such as lead, cadmium and mineral hydrocarbons in food are controlled by regulations under the Health Act, 1947.[23]

Control of Sale of Drugs, Medicines and Poisons

Poisons

The Poisons (Ireland) Act, 1870, the Pharmacy Act (Ireland), 1875 (and the amending Act of 1890) and the Arsenic Act, 1851 provide, *inter alia,* that certain scheduled poisons may be sold only by qualified persons, i.e. registered pharmaceutical chemists, etc. and that certain poisons may be sold only to persons known to the seller. All scheduled poisons must be labelled according to the provisions of the Acts.

Regulations under the Poisons Act, 1961, are at present in course of preparation. These Regulations will provide an up to date code for controlling the sale and distribution of a wide range of substances, which will replace the provisions of earlier enactments.

The Poisons Act, 1961 (Paraquat) Regulations, 1975, impose certain restrictions on the sale and distribution of paraquat and specify certain requirements as to packaging, labelling and record-keeping.

Medical preparations

Under the Medical Preparations (Control of Sale) Regulations, 1966 (as amended by the 1971 and 1976 Regulations) certain scheduled substances and preparations may be sold by retail only by pharmaceutical chemists and other qualified persons.

---

[22]The Food Standards Act, 1974, was co-sponsored by the Minister for Health, the Minister for Agriculture and Fisheries and the Minister for Industry and Commerce 'to enable standards for human food to be established and enforced and to provide for related matters'.

[23]See list in Appendix J.

In addition certain substances and preparations may be sold only on prescription. The substances covered by the regulations include antibiotics, certain drugs acting on the central nervous system and hormone preparations.

The Medical Preparations (Control of Amphetamine) Regulations, 1969 (as amended by the 1970 Regulations) prohibit generally the manufacture, importation, sale and distribution of preparations containing amphetamines and their derivatives. The regulations contain provisions enabling the Minister for Health to grant a licence permitting the manufacture, importation, distribution or sale of a preparation covered by the regulations, subject to compliance with certain conditions.

The Medical Preparations (Advertisement and Sale) Regulations 1958, provide that medical preparations may not be publicly advertised in a manner that might lead to their use in the diagnosis, prevention or treatment in humans of certain scheduled ailments (e.g. cancer, tuberculosis, diabetes, etc.) and that all medical preparations on retail sale must contain a statement on the label or container thereof showing their exact contents.

The advertisement of cures for venereal disease is prohibited by the Venereal Disease Act, 1917.

Safety, quality and efficacy of medicines
The Therapeutic Substances Act, 1932, applies to vaccines, sera, toxins, antitoxins, antigens and certain other substances, whether used in the treatment of human or animal disease. The general purpose of the Act is to ensure that such substances, the purity and potency of which cannot be adequately tested by chemical means, will comply with certain standards of potency, quality and purity. The controls provide for the licensing of manufacture and importation; the sale of such substances is subject to requirements regarding type of container, labelling and compliance with certain conditions as to expiry dates, etc.

The European Communities (Proprietary Medicinal Products) Regulations, 1975 require that new proprietary medicinal products may not be placed on the market after 1 April 1976, unless they comply with the provisions of EEC Council Directives 65/65, 73/318 and 75/319. The regulations also provide for the progressive application of the requirements of those

Directives to proprietary medicinal products which were already on the market on 1 October 1974.

The Medical Preparations (Licensing of Manufacture) Regulations, 1974 (as amended by the 1975 Regulations) and the Medical Preparations (Wholesale Licences) Regulations, 1974 prohibit respectively the manufacture, and sale by wholesale, of any medical preparation for human use except in accordance with a licence granted by the Minister for Health.

The Pharmacopoeia Act, 1931, provides that any medicines of the Irish Pharmacopoeia may be compounded only in accordance with the formularies of such Pharmacopoeia. Under an amendment contained in the Misuse of Drugs Act, 1977, there is provision for compliance with the standards and monographs of the European Pharmacopoeia.

Prevention of Drug Abuse, Illicit Traffic, etc.

The Dangereous Drugs Act, 1934 and the regulations made thereunder regulated and controlled the production, supply and possession of narcotic drugs such as opiates and cocaine, as well as cannabis and a range of synthetic opiates such as pethidine, methadone, etc. The purpose of the Act was to prevent illicit traffic in and abuse of those drugs and to give effect to the international conventions prepared for that purpose.

The 1934 Act and regulations were recently replaced by the Misuse of Drugs Act, 1977, which extends control to a wider range of substances, provides a more flexible control structure and more extensive powers for dealing with various drug offences and persons who become involved in the abuse of drugs.

The Health (Possession of Controlled Substances) Regulations, 1970 make it an offence to be in possession of certain scheduled substances except in circumstances specified in the regulations, such as possession by a doctor, dentist or pharmacist for the purpose of his profession, or where a person obtains the substance on a prescription for medical or dental treatment. The substances covered by the regulations are amphetamines and similar substances, barbiturates and other hypnotics, and synthetic hallucinogenic substances such as lysergic acid diethylamide (L.S.D.). These regulations are also to be replaced by new controls under the Misuse of Drugs Act, 1977.

The General Medical Service

Administration

The health boards are responsible for the arrangements for the provision of general medical services under the choice of doctor scheme. Participating doctors and pharmacists enter into agreement with the boards. The General Medical Services (Payments) Board which is a joint body of health boards established under section II of the Health Act, 1970 is responsible for the calculation and making of payments to both doctors and pharmacists who participate in the service.

PART I

The Participation of Medical Practitioners

General conditions

1. The conditions for participation in the service are specified in the agreement, which is in a prescribed form, between the health board and the medical practitioner.

2. The conditions for participation in the service (including fees) which have been agreed on between the Minister for Health and the Irish Medical Association and the Medical Union relate only to a situation in which there is no significant change in the percentage of population eligible for the service.

Choice of doctor

3. Subject to what follows and to paragraph 6 below, an eligible person is allowed to register with any participating doctor who has not already got a list up to the maximum (see paragraph 10 below). His choice is, however, subject to the condition that the doctor does not live more than seven miles from the patient, but this condition does not apply in certain individual cases, such as where there is no doctor within seven miles of the patient. Where the doctor wishes to take on a patient living more than seven miles from him and where other doctors practise within seven miles of the patient's residence, the domiciliary fee

payable is that appropriate to a distance of seven miles.

Persons for whom doctor is responsible
4. The doctor is responsible for
(a) all eligible persons whom he has accepted for inclusion in his list and who have not been notified to him by the board as having ceased to be on the list;
(b) all eligible persons assigned to him by the board in accordance with paragraph 5 hereunder and who have not been notified to him by the board as having ceased to be on his list;
(c) all eligible persons whom he has accepted as temporary residents;
(d) all eligible persons in respect of whom he is acting as deputy to another practitioner;
(e) all eligible persons whom it is necessary for him to treat in an emergency situation.
5. The doctor may be assigned eligible persons by the board. In areas where there is a choice between doctors providing services for eligible persons the power of assignment by the board is used only in the case of persons who have unsuccessfully applied to a number of doctors for acceptance on their lists. The assignment of a patient is to the nearest doctor unless there is a valid contraindication, but assignments are reviewed at reasonable intervals. In areas where the choice of another doctor is impossible or impracticable, the doctor is obliged to accept on his list all eligible patients in that area who seek inclusion in his list. In the exceptional case where a group of patients more than ten miles from a doctor is assigned to him there is a special allowance for this responsibility in addition to the scheduled fees. The amount of the allowance is related to the number of patients and the distance involved and is negotiated with the two medical organisations.
6. The doctor is not required to provide services for any person whom he is unwilling to accept as a patient unless the person concerned is one assigned to him by the board or unless he is called upon to attend the patient in an emergency situation.

Temporary residents
7. A temporary resident is an eligible person who temporarily moves into a district not served by the doctor in whose list he is

included and who does not, at the time of his arrival in the district, intend to remain there for a period exceeding three months. If his stay within the district extends to more than three months, his residence shall as from the end of that period cease to be regarded as temporary.

Itinerant families

8. Health boards, through their own officers or through voluntary organisations, ensure that eligible itinerant families are issued with medical cards and are accepted on the lists of doctors in the areas where the itinerants are normally resident. Where itinerant families move outside these areas they are regarded as temporary residents.

Unregistered children

9. Where a doctor is requested to provide a service for a young child whose name has not already been added to the list of dependants covered by the family registration, he shall provide the service and claim the appropriate fee on a specially prescribed form.

Limitation on numbers

10. The normal limit to the number of eligible persons on the doctor's list is 2,000 but in exceptional cases, the board may decide not to apply this limit.

Discontinuance of acceptance of a person

11. A doctor wishing to discontinue his acceptance of an eligible person, other than a person assigned by the board, may do so on giving notice to the board. If the doctor informs the board of his desire to discontinue his acceptance of an eligible person, the board notifies the person accordingly and supplies him with a notice enabling him to apply to another doctor. The person's name is removed from the doctor's list as from the date on which the doctor receives intimation that the person has been accepted by or assigned to another doctor.

Change of doctor

12. Where a person whose name is included in the list of a doctor wishes to transfer to the list of another doctor he applies on

a prescribed form to the health board seeking such transfer. The name of the other doctor is specified in the application and it is a matter for the person to seek from him acceptance of the transfer and for the doctor to indicate such acceptance on the application form. The first doctor ceases to be responsible for the patient on the date he receives a notification from the health board that the patient has been transferred to another list.

Manner of providing service

13. The doctor is obliged to render to his patients all proper and necessary treatment of a kind usually undertaken by a general medical practitioner and not requiring special skill or experience of a degree or kind which general practitioners cannot reasonably be expected to possess.

14. The doctor undertakes to be available for consultation at his surgery (surgeries) for a specified number of hours weekly and to be available for consultation and for domiciliary visiting for an aggregate of forty hours weekly during normal hours. He also undertakes to have suitable arrangements to enable contact with him outside normal hours for emergency cases.

15. Where a doctor chooses to arrange some routine surgery hours or to do some of his routine domiciliary calls outside normal working hours he is not entitled to claim more than the normal fee for these services.

16. The doctor undertakes to maintain his surgery (surgeries) in a suitable condition for the purposes of his medical practice and, if required, to allow inspection by a representative of the board for the purposes of establishing its (their) suitability.

17. Surgery arrangements made by the doctor may not discriminate between eligible persons and the practitioner's private patients.

Obtaining consultant advice

18. Subject to such conditions or directions as the Minister for Health may lay down from time to time following consultation with the medical organisations a doctor may when he considers it desirable have a consultation with another medical practitioner in regard to an eligible patient on his list and the health board is liable for the cost of such consultation.

Prescribing and dispensing

19. The doctor is obliged to prescribe on the official prescription form such drugs and appliances as he considers necessary for the eligible person and in doing so he must act in accordance with any administrative requirements as to the completion of the form. While nothing in these requirements may interfere with the practitioner's discretion as to the amount and nature of the items prescribed, it is expected that doctors will bear in mind the need for economy. Where the prescribing pattern of a medical practitioner appears to be abnormal the circumstances may be investigated by a medical officer acting on behalf of the General Medical Services (Payments) Board. If the medical officer so decides the circumstances may then be referred for consideration by an investigating committee referred to in paragraph 56.

20. The doctor shall supply to a person on his list such drugs and appliances as the doctor shall consider necessary for immediate administration or application. Where the doctor is not a dispensing doctor he may recoup from a retail pharmacist who has an agreement with the health board, the items so supplied by giving to him on the prescribed form a 'prescription' in the name of the patient or patients.

21. Subject to paragraphs 22 and 25, dispensing under the scheme is normally done by a retail pharmacist.

22. Where a doctor has only one centre of practice and it is three miles or more from the nearest retail pharmacist all patients on the doctor's list are asked to indicate whether they wish to have their prescriptions dispensed by the doctor or by a retail pharmacist. To remunerate him for his services a doctor is paid an annual fee in respect of each patient who opts to have his prescriptions dispensed by the doctor.

23. Where a doctor has a number of centres of practice, one or more within three miles of a pharmacy and one or more over three miles from a pharmacy only those patients who would normally be expected to attend the distant centre have a right to opt for dispensing by the doctor.

24. When a pharmacist opens a pharmacy within three miles of a dispensing doctor's centre of practice his eligible patients cease to have a choice between the doctor and the pharmacist for dispensing purposes. As from a date to be determined by

the health board these patients may have their prescriptions dispensed by the pharmacist (subject to paragraph 25).

25. Where a doctor lives within three miles of a pharmacist but where in the view of the health board it would be a hardship on certain individual patients because of disability to obtain their prescriptions from a retail pharmacist the doctor may, in such instances, be required to dispense for the patients. The doctor is paid an annual dispensing fee for each of these patients.

26. A dispensing doctor is obliged to obtain his requirements of drugs for eligible persons from a pharmacist(s) who has (have) entered into an agreement with the health board, and to complete requisitions, returns of stock and such other records as may be required of him. The pharmacist would be one in the doctor's normal area of practice or, if there was none in that area, a reasonably convenient pharmacist outside that area.

27. An eligible person receiving consultant out-patient care at a hospital is normally referred back to his general practitioner who issues him with a prescription for whatever medicines he may require. In the exceptional instance where the hospital doctor considers it essential that he should issue a prescription himself a sufficient quantity may be dispensed from hospital stocks to carry the patient over until he can attend his general practitioner.

Medical records

28. A doctor is obliged to comply with such directions or regulations as the Minister for Health may make from time to time after consultation with the medical profession in regard to the keeping of medical records.

29. When an eligible patient for whom the doctor has been responsible is transferred to the list of another doctor providing services under Section 58 of the Health Act, 1970, the former doctor, subject to the consent of the patient, gives to the latter doctor a summary of the medical history and condition of the patient.

Rights of participation by doctors

30. On the commencement of the re-organised service the following categories of general practitioner had automatic right of entry to the scheme provided they had not reached 70 years

of age:

(a) Permanent district medical officers from their then centres of practice.

(b) Temporary district medical officers with at least two years' continuous temporary service in one or more districts from the centres of practice where they were practising on the date of the commencement of the new service in their areas.

(c) Any doctor who has been in private general practice in an area for two years prior to the commencement of the scheme in that area, from the centre or centres from which he has practised for at least two years.

(d) Any doctor who having completed two years' service in hospital or general practice after the completion of his intern year had set up practice before 17 July 1970 in respect of the centre(s) in which he was then in practice.

31. In addition to the foregoing a health board could in the light of the need of the area admit to the scheme at its commencement other practitioners in practice in the area.

Vacancies in the service

32. Normally vacancies are filled by the health board following public advertisement and interview.

33. In 1975 certain changes in the arrangements for filling vacancies were introduced. These provided for the admission to the general medical service doctors in the following categories subject to certain conditions:

(a) any doctor who had been in general practice for at least two years prior to 1 October 1974;

(b) any single handed general practitioner not covered by (a) in practice on 1 October 1974 when he had completed two years in general practice;

(c) any partner as on 1 October 1974 of a doctor or doctors already participating in the scheme.

(d) any doctor who was on 1 October 1974 employed as assistant to a doctor in the scheme or who is admitted under (a) and who became a partner of such a doctor prior to 31 December 1975 or six months after the date of the Agreement on the document, whichever is the later.

34. While in relation to future vacancies the main method of entry to the scheme would continue to be by open competition

measures to encourage the creation of partnerships and group practices were introduced. These are outlined in paragraphs 35 to 38 hereunder.

35. The creation of a position as partner, or as an additional member of a group practice, or as an assistant with a view to partnership for the purpose of the general medical service, is subject to the approval of the health board. In considering any such proposal the board has regard to the total practice of the applicant. Before giving approval the board must be satisfied:—
(a) that the creation of the position is preferable to the creation of an additional position which could be filled by open competition in the normal way; and
(b) that the creation of the position will not result in the admission of a particular person into the general medical service while other equally well or better qualified persons are not given a reasonable chance to compete. Where the chief executive officer proposes to seek the approval of the board to the creation of a position as a partner, or as an additional member of a group practice, or as an assistant with a view to partnership he shall, before doing so, consult the medical organisations.

36. Where a health board agrees to the creation of a partnership or an addition to a group practice or to the recruitment of an assistant with a view to a partnership the position is advertised in the normal way but the doctor or doctors involved or a nominee of the doctor or doctors involved in the proposed taking in of a partner, or additional member or assistant is entitled to sit on the selection board. The selection board is obliged to pay due regard to any objection of this representative to the giving of the post to a particular individual or individuals. If the board considers it desirable it may not recommend any candidate for appointment.

Employment of an assistant with a view to partnership
37. Where the health board has agreed to the recruitment of an assistant with a view to partnership the following provisions apply:—
(a) the doctor recommended by the selection board shall serve as an assistant for a trial period of six months. The arrangement may be terminated by either party, or by mutual agree-

ment, at any time during this period;

(b) if the arrangement is terminated a further recommendation of an assistant may be made by a selection board constituted in accordance with paragraph 36 but if a partnership is not created within two years of the first assistant taking up duty the agreement of the health board to the employment of an assistant with a view to partnership in the general medical service shall lapse;

(c) during the trial period an assistant is not entitled to enter into an agreement with the health board to provide services for eligible patients. He may, on behalf of the participating doctor, provide services for such patients but he shall not be assigned sole responsibility for any specific patients or group of patients;

(d) the participating doctor shall retain responsibility for the provision of services for all patients on his list and shall also be generally responsible for the visiting and prescribing patterns of the assistant;

(e) after entering into partnership at the conclusion of the trial period the assistant shall be entitled to enter into an agreement with the health board to provide services for eligible patients as a member of the partnership.

Employment of other assistants

38. Where an assistant (other than that referred to in the preceding paragraph) is employed the doctor has to notify the health board to this effect and the following provisions apply:

(a) such an assistant has no right of succession to the general medical service panel,

(b) the participating doctor must normally provide, in person, services in accordance with the provisions of his contract,

(c) such an assistant could deal with general medical service patients as locum and he could also deal with such patients when it is not practicable for the participating doctor to provide the services in person, but there can be no assignment to the assistant of any specific patients or group of patients,

(d) the participating doctor would retain full responsibility for the proper care of all patients on his list,

(e) the participating doctor would be responsible for the visiting and prescribing patterns of the assistant. The selection of an assistant would normally be a matter for the participating doctor or doctors.

39. In addition to the foregoing any doctor established in his own right in private practice in a particular centre for seven years can become entitled to take public patients (but would not, of course, be given any guaranteed panel of such patients). Such a doctor would be entitled to apply to the health board for entry into the scheme and if he satisfies the board that he complied with the provision mentioned, he would normally be admitted to the scheme.

40. While the permanent filling of a vacancy is pending, transfers of patients from the list for the vacant practice are not allowed. On a practitioner taking up duty to fill a vacancy, he has assigned to him his predecessor's list of eligible persons, but any person on that list may subsequently exercise his normal right to transfer to another participating practitioner. Unless there are exceptional circumstances this right may not be exercised until three months have expired from the date on which the doctor takes up duty.

41. While the vacancy exists, the health board may fill it in a temporary capacity or may assign patients on a temporary basis to other participating practitioners but the health board must without undue delay take steps to fill the post in a permanent capacity, if it is to be filled. The number of patients assigned on a temporary basis would be subject to the normal limit referred to in paragraph 10.

Qualifications

42. The Minister may after consultation with the medical profession prescribe minimum qualifications and experience for applicants for vacancies.

Irish language

43. As has been the case of the dispensary service it is a condition for participation in the service in a Gaeltacht area that a doctor has a satisfactory knowledge of the Irish language.

Age limit

44. The contract of a participating doctor ceases to operate on his reaching 70 years of age.

Locums

45. The doctor makes arrangements for the employment of a suitably qualified deputy during absences. The initial obligation to obtain a locum rests with the participating doctor but health boards co-operate in obtaining one. Where a doctor falls ill the health board, if requested, has the obligation to obtain a locum.

The payment of the deputy is a matter for the doctor unless it is the board's responsibility to make such payment. A participating doctor, other than a district medical officer who has rights in connection with locums, gets an allowance of £186 per annum as a contribution towards locum and other practice expenses.

Partnerships and group practice

46. Where two or more doctors proposing to enter into agreements with the board are in partnership or in group practice each has to enter into an individual agreement with the board and will have his individual list of eligible patients and will be responsible for them in the same way as if he were practising independently.

47. Where one partner or one member of a group practice provides treatment for an eligible person on another partner's list, he will do so in the capacity of a locum tenens and he will not be entitled to claim an emergency fee or a temporary resident's fee for attending such a person.

Remuneration

48. The doctor may not demand or accept any fee or other remuneration for services rendered under Section 58 of the Health Act, 1970 other than the payments prescribed from time to time by the Minister for Health.

49. As from 1 November 1977 the scale of fees payable to participating practitioners was as follows:

Surgery Consultations	£
(a) Normal hours	1.48
(b) outside normal hours, other than (c)	2.11
(c) midnight to 8 a.m.	4.19

Domiciliary Consultations
(a) normal hours urban

up to 3 miles	2.21
3-5 miles	2.86
5-7 miles	3.87
7-10 miles	4.84
over 10 miles	6.05

(b) outside normal hours other than (c) urban

up to 3 miles	2.86
3-5 miles	3.72
5-7 miles	4.84
7-10 miles	6.42
over 10 miles	7.56

(c) midnight to 8 a.m. urban

up to 3 miles	5.64
3-5 miles	7.24
5-7 miles	9.18
7-10 miles	10.22
over 10 miles	11.24
Emergency fee	1.63
Dispensing fee	1.63
Rural practitioners allowance	960.00
Sessional Rates—Homes for Aged	9.96

50. Where a doctor attends to more than one eligible patient in a household in the course of a domiciliary visit a fee at the appropriate domiciliary rate is payable for the first patient and a fee at the appropriate surgery rate for the other patient(s).

51. Where a doctor provides services from more than one centre of practice his fee for a domiciliary service is related to the distance the patient lives from the doctor's main centre of practice.

52. Where a doctor attends eligible persons in a home for the aged fees are payable on a sessional basis for routine visiting at the rate of £9.96 per three hour session. The amount due to a doctor is calculated by totalling the number of hours spent by him each month in the routine visiting of eligible patients. The appropriate domiciliary fee is payable for non-routine calls to the home.

53. Where a doctor undertakes an urgent visit between 11 p.m.

and midnight which necessarily involves his remaining on the call until after midnight he may claim the appropriate after-midnight fee for the service.

Medical certificates

54. The fees payable to the doctor cover the issue by him of certificates for such purposes as may be prescribed by the Minister for Health after consultation with the medical profession.

Submission and processing of claims for fees

55. As stated in the preamble a special central unit has been set up to pay accounts submitted by doctors and pharmacists under the scheme. The claim forms used by doctors are prescribed after agreement with the medical organisations and are so designed as to minimise the clerical work to be done by the doctor. In regard to each service the doctor's claim shows the patient's number, the type of visit (domiciliary or surgery) and whether the visit was during or outside normal hours. Special claim forms have to be completed for services to temporary residents; to unregistered children in a family covered by a medical card; for emergency services to eligible persons not on the doctor's list and for routine visits to homes for the aged. Payments are processed by computer.

56. The computer maintains a continuing record of a doctor's visiting pattern. Where an instance of abnormal consultation is revealed the medical officer attached to the central unit seeks clarification from the doctor concerned. If there is evidence to suggest that the rate of consultation was not justified the medical officer reports the facts to an investigating committee consisting of a nominee of the Minister, a representative of the organised profession and the medical officer acting on behalf of the central unit (not being the medical officer who investigated the circumstances).

57. The investigating committee decides whether the instance calls for no further action, for a warning, for a reduction in fees claimed or, in a serious case, for referral to the disciplinary tribunal referred to in paragraph 77. It is open to a doctor to appeal to the disciplinary tribunal against a decision of the committee. The form of agreement which doctors enter into with health boards includes a more detailed description of the

provisions for penalties and the reduction of fees.

Practice payments for remote areas

58. These areas are specified from time to time, as required, by the Minister in consultation with the health boards and the medical organisations. They include extremely remote areas such as the islands and some mainland districts which call for special consideration.

59. In these areas the doctor may opt for full fees *or* the existing special salary which is currently paid for such areas (£6,600) *or* the normal district medical officer salary scale (£3,910–£5,339) plus half fees. Depending on circumstances the health board may permit entry to the scale above the minimum in the case of a doctor opting for the third method of payment.

Practice payments for other rural areas

60. Where a doctor lives and practises in a centre with a population of less than 500 and where there is not a town with a population of 1,500 or more within a three-mile radius of that centre the doctor is entitled to special rural practice concessions.

61. In these areas the doctor is paid full fees. In addition a rural practice allowance of £960 a year is payable:

(a) to a district medical officer with guarantees who opts to be paid on a fee basis,

(b) to any other participating practitioner who, at the commencement of the scheme, is entitled to participate in it and who is the sole participating practitioner in the centre in question,

(c) to any other participating practitioner if the health board decide to make this payment to retain him in the area.

62. Where a district medical officer has guarantees, he is entitled to the fees plus the allowance of £960 *or* the current salary for his existing post, whichever is the greater.

Practice premises—standards

63. It is a condition of the practitioner's contract that on entry or by a specified date he has suitable premises available for his practice in which there will be common access to him by his

eligible and private patients.

64. A health board requires a participating doctor to provide and to continue to maintain the following facilities for his patients:

(a) a waiting room with a reasonable standard of comfort, sufficient in size to accommodate the normal demands of his practice for both eligible and private patients and with adequate seating accommodation;

(b) a surgery sufficient in size for the requirements of normal general practice. Its facilities should include electric light, hot and cold running water, an examination couch and other essential needs of general practice;

(c) a telephone should be available for the doctor on the premises at the main centre of practice;

(d) toilet facilities should be accessible to patients.

65. A doctor is expected by the health board to give facilities for inspection of premises to establish suitability.

Practice premises—grants for improvements

66. Health boards are empowered to give grants towards the provision of new practice premises or for the improvement or extension of the existing practice premises of participating doctors.

67. Application is made to the health board which considers whether it should give a grant in the light of

(a) the number of eligible persons on the practitioner's list,

(b) the extent and nature of the accommodation already available to him in his practice premises and

(c) the availability of alternative facilities for general practitioners under the control of the health board.

68. The additional accommodation in respect of which a grant may be given is related to the extent and standard considered necessary by the health board to allow the practitioner to provide in a reasonable manner for all his patients. If the practitioner provides more accommodation than is considered essential or provides accommodation of a standard higher than necessary, the additional expenditure is entirely his own responsibility.

69. In the case of an individual participating practitioner a health board may give a grant amounting to 25 per cent of the

cost of the approved works subject to a maximum of £1,000. The health board may, however, give a grant amounting to $37\frac{1}{2}$ per cent subject to a maximum of £1,500 to an individual participating practitioner in a 'remote' area or 'other rural' area (as defined in paragraph 60).

70. In the case of two participating practitioners operating in association from the same premises a health board may give a grant amounting to $37\frac{1}{2}$ per cent of the cost of the approved works subject to a maximum of £1,500.

71. In the case of group practices a health board may give grants of 50 per cent of the cost of the approved works subject to a maximum of £2,000 for three doctors, increasing by £500 in respect of each additional doctor in the practice.

72. A health board may require a practitioner who has received a grant to recoup all or portion of it should he voluntarily cease to participate in the scheme within three years of the payment of the grant.

Practice premises—use of official premises

73. Participating doctors may be offered facilities to practise in existing health centres, dispensaries or other health board accommodation. Where a permanent district medical officer occupies a dispensary residence he is allowed to continue in occupation as long as he participates in the new service in the area concerned. Where a dispensary and residence are sited together only the doctor occupying the residence has a right to use that dispensary.

74. No charge is made to a dispensary doctor with automatic right of participation, using a health centre, dispensary or other health board premises. An appropriate negotiated contribution towards running expenses is made by other practitioners availing of such facilities but they are provided free of charge for approved partnerships or group practices.

Complaints against doctors

75. Complaints on the provision (or non-provision) of services by doctors are investigated in the first placed by the staff of the health board. If the chief executive officer of the health board decides that a complaint is unfounded no further action is taken. If he decides that it is well-founded but relatively trivial,

he has power to communicate with the doctor on the subject matter of the complaint.

76. If the complaint appears on preliminary investigation to be of a serious nature the chief executive officer shall refer it to the Disciplinary Tribunal.[1]

77. The Disciplinary Tribunal is a special statutory body appointed by the Minister to deal with such complaints. It consists of a chairman selected in agreement with the medical profession and an even number of other members, of whom half are doctors appointed from a panel agreed with the profession.

78. The Tribunal, having considered the complaint with all practicable speed may either:—

(a) dismiss it and let this dismissal be known to all concerned;

(b) uphold it and direct termination of the doctor's agreement;

(c) uphold it but recommend a lesser penalty by way of deduction of a specified sum from the doctor's remuneration or

(d) uphold it but decide that it is sufficient to admonish the doctor for his conduct.

79. There is an appeal to the Minister against the termination of an agreement or other penalty recommended by the Tribunal. On such an appeal the Minister may uphold, modify or reverse the decision of the Tribunal. This in no way cuts across normal rights of recourse to the courts.

Termination of agreement

80. A doctor may terminate his agreement on giving three months' notice, or such shorter notice as may be acceptable to the board.

81. The agreement shall be terminated forthwith where the medical practitioner's name is removed from the register of medical practitioners maintained by the Medical Registration Council of Ireland or where the disciplinary tribunal established to deal with complaints against medical practitioners participating in the service has so directed and after appeal, where made, the Minister for Health or the Courts have upheld the decision.

82. The agreement shall be terminated on a doctor's taking up

[1]Established under article 8 of Health Services Regulations, 1972 (S.I. No. 88).

wholetime employment outside the service.

83. The board may terminate the agreement where:—

(a) the medical practitioner ceases to comply with the terms of the agreement, or

(b) the medical practitioner has been certified in accordance with a prescribed procedure to be discussed with the medical organisations to be suffering from permanent infirmity of mind or body.

84. An appeal lies to the Minister for Health against the board's decision to terminate the agreement and the doctor also has a right of appeal to the Courts.

PART II

Supply of Drugs, Medicines and Appliances

Dispensing by pharmacists
1. The dispensing of drugs and medicines for an eligible person in the re-organised general medical service is normally done by a contracting pharmacist. The word pharmacist throughout means a registered pharmaceutical chemist or a registered dispensing chemist and druggist lawfully 'keeping open shop' in accordance with the provisions of the Pharmacy Acts 1875-1962.
2. When a pharmacist receives a prescription on an official form signed by a doctor he dispenses the items listed on the form. The items dispensed by the pharmacist should be entirely in accordance with the doctor's prescription unless the prescription contains obvious errors or omissions.

General conditions for participation of retail pharmacists
3. Every retail pharmacist is eligible for participation in the scheme provided he enters into the prescribed agreement with the relevant health board or health boards.
4. The form of agreement between the pharmacist and the health board was the subject of discussion between the Department of Health and the Joint Negotiating Committee representing community pharmacists. In general the provisions of the agreement are based on the terms contained herein.
5. A pharmacist's agreement with a health board may be terminated by the board where it is satisfied that the pharmacist has failed to observe the terms of the agreement or that the pharmacist has been convicted of a criminal offence relating to the practice of pharmacy. The pharmacist may appeal to the Minister for Health against this termination.
6. A pharmacist's agreement with a health board shall automatically terminate upon the removal of his name from the register of the Pharmaceutical Society of Ireland.
7. A pharmacist may terminate his agreement on giving three months notice or such shorter notice as may be acceptable to the health board.

8. The conditions (including fees) for participation in the service which have been agreed on between the Minister for Health and the Joint Negotiating Committee relate only to a situation in which there will be no significant change in the percentage of population now eligible for the service.

Premises

9. A pharmacist is required to maintain satisfactory premises, equipment and stock and in this respect the premises may be inspected by an officer of the health board or of the central pricing agency.

Hours of business

10. The pharmacist is obliged to keep his premises open for dispensing prescriptions during the hours specified in his agreement with the health board.

Basis of remuneration

11. The pharmacist is remunerated on the basis of the recoupment to him of the ingredient cost of prescription items dispensed for eligible patients under the scheme together with a fee for each item. The fee contains specific elements to cover the cost of containers, capital investment and obsolescence. Higher fees are paid for extemporaneous prescribing and for prescription items which involve the fitting of appliances. An additional fee is payable for urgent prescriptions dispensed outside contract hours.

12. The price of a proprietary item to the pharmacist is taken as the basic ex-wholesale price ruling during the month the prescription was dispensed. The ingredient cost of non-proprietary items is arrived at on the basis of lists agreed between the Department of Health and the Joint Negotiating Committee. A tariff is circulated to all pharmacists detailing the rates which are payable in respect of non-proprietary drugs, medicines and appliances. Amendments to the tariff are circulated from time to time as necessary. The tariff does not contain the prices of proprietary items. Manufacturing and wholesale firms notify the General Medical Services (Payments) Board of price changes in goods in advance of implementation.

Details of remuneration
13. The scale of fees payable to pharmacists at 1 November 1977 is as follows:—

Fee	Pence
Basic fee	50.64
Extemporaneous compounding	101.28
Measuring and fitting	151.92
Dressings	
for up to 3 items on a form	
for 4 to 6 items on a form	
(pro rata increase for additional items)	
Urgent fee and late fee	142.23
Midnight to 8 a.m. (resident)	172.05
Midnight to 8 a.m. (non-resident)	294.53

14. *Supplies to dispensing doctors:* Pharmacists supplying dispensing doctors are reimbursed on the basis of the basic ex-wholesale price, with the addition of 25 per cent on cost.

15. *Advance payments:* On the submission of the first claim by a pharmacist participating in the scheme, an advance payment within three weeks is made to him on the basis of £1 for each of the estimated number of prescription items in his claim. The claim is paid in full within a further 30 days but the pharmacist will continue to retain the original advance payment as an advance for subsequent claims. In the event of the pharmacist leaving the scheme, this advance payment is repayable by him.

16. If, after the scheme has been in operation for six months, the original advance payment is shown to be less, by more than 20%, than the monthly average payment, an appropriate adjustment in the advance payment is made.

17. If the original advance payment is shown to have been too large in the light of the subsequent monthly claims of the pharmacist, the General Medical Services (Payments) Board makes an appropriate deduction from payments due to the pharmacist.

18. *Value added tax:* Pharmacists are recouped in full value added tax paid by them in respect of services given under this scheme.

19. *Allowances for obsolescence, capital investment and containers:* The basic fee contains an element of 7p to recoup the

pharmacist for the cost of obsolescence, capital investment and containers.

Provisions regarding packs and containers
20. *Pack sizes:* The size of pack from which pharmacists are expected to dispense prescriptions under the scheme is the size which would normally have a shelf life of one month having regard to the volume of business of the particular pharmacist.
21. Where it appears that a pharmacist is dispensing from a smaller pack than is necessary and thereby increasing the ingredient cost of the item, the General Medical Services (Payments) Board seeks an explanation from the pharmacist and may make an appropriate deduction from payments due to him.
22. Where, in order to meet the requirements of a particularly expensive prescription, a pharmacist is obliged to purchase a larger quantity than prescribed and where portion of that pack remains on his hands after an agreed period, the full cost of the pack is paid to the pharmacist and the balance of the pack may be taken into stock by a health board pharmacy.
23. *Container standards:* Capsules, tablets, etc. should be dispensed in their original packs or in rigid containers. Containers made from paper board material are not acceptable.

Procedure for submission of claims for remuneration
24. A code book (with detailed instructions) covering drugs, medicines, dressings and appliances in common use has been issued to each pharmacist. When a pharmacist dispenses a prescription he has to insert on the prescription form the appropriate code number for each item dispensed. He also stamps and retains the form, which is in duplicate.
25. If the prescription has been marked urgent by the doctor or certified urgent by the pharmacist and has been submitted to and dispensed by the pharmacist outside contract hours, he endorses it with the time of dispensing.
26. It is essential that the number of the patient should have been entered on the prescription form by the doctor. A prescription without the patient's number cannot be processed.
27. A pharmacist forwards all prescriptions dispensed by him under the scheme during a calendar month to reach the

General Medical Services (Payments) Board not later than the 7th day of the following month. The period is extended to take account of any public holidays. The pharmacist retains the duplicates of the prescriptions.

28. Before submitting the prescriptions to the General Medical Services (Payments) Board, the pharmacist sorts each bundle of forms into the following categories:—

(a) forms with all items coded,

(b) forms with some items coded,

(c) forms with no items coded,

(d) stock orders from dispensing doctors,

(e) forms for the previous month which were returned to the pharmacist for clarification,

(f) forms for which an urgent fee is claimed.

29. The pharmacist must also complete a simple covering duplicate form which indicates the pharmacist's name and address and the number of forms in each category.

30. Each pharmacist receives an acknowledgement of the receipt of his bundle and he is also informed if no bundle is received from him.

31. Payment to the pharmacist is normally made in full during the second half of the month following that in which the prescriptions are submitted.

32. Where it is found that a prescription has been issued in error by a doctor to a person not eligible for participation in the scheme and the pharmacist has *bona fide* fulfilled the terms of the prescription, he is paid the appropriate amount for it.

33. Each pharmacist receives with his payment cheque a detailed statement showing the manner in which the payment was calculated.

APPENDIX H

Summary of Provisions on Mental Treatment

This is a brief summary of the contents of the law on reception, etc., of psychiatric patients. In no sense is it a complete statement of that law. This is basically contained in the Mental Treatment Act, 1945 but that Act has been amended and adapted on several occasions. The provisions in it on administration and eligibility have been superseded by the Health Acts and the 1945 Act was otherwise amended in 1953 and 1961. New Regulations under the Act were made in the latter year. The law as it stood in 1961 was set out in a booklet entitled 'Mental Treatment Acts, 1945 to 1961: statutory provisions, regulations and explanatory notes regarding the reception, treatment, detention and discharge of mentally ill patients'—which was published by the Stationery Office. Several technical adaptations in the provisions as they stood at that time were made by the Mental Treatment Acts (Adaptation) Order, 1971, to bring those provisions into conformity with the administrative changes effected by the Health Act, 1970.

Modes of admission to mental hospitals
There are three categories in mental hospitals—voluntary patients, temporary patients and those certified as persons of unsound mind.

Reception orders for persons of unsound mind[1]
An application to have a person received as being of unsound mind in a mental hospital is normally made by the husband, wife or other relative. Where the patient is in one of the classes entitled to use the health board's service and it is desired to have him admitted as such to the district mental hospital, the application is made to a medical practitioner. He examines the patient and, if satisfied, recommends that he be received in the district mental hospital.

[1]Sections 162 to 183 of 1945 Act (as amended and adapted) and Part V of the Mental Treatment Regulations, 1961.

231

Where such a recommendation has been made, the patient may then be brought (with the assistance of an escort from the Garda Síochána if required for the safe conveyance of the patient) to the district mental hospital. The health board may co-operate with the applicant in making arrangements for the removal of the person to hospital. The person is then examined by the medical officer in charge or a deputy. If that officer is satisfied that the person should be received, he makes an 'eligible patient reception order'. This authorises the patient's detention in the mental hospital 'until his removal or discharge by proper authority or his death'.

Where the person is to be admitted as a private patient, whether to a district mental hospital or another mental hospital, the husband, wife or other relative may apply to any medical practitioner for 'a private patient reception order'. That medical practitioner arranges with a second medical practitioner to examine the patient separately and if both doctors are satisfied that it should be done, they make the reception order. This authorises the person in charge of the institution named in the order to receive and detain the patient.

Temporary patients[2]
Mental hospitals and homes which are approved for that purpose by the Minister for Health may receive temporary patients. The admission and reception of such patients is governed by procedures similar to those for persons of unsound mind but the detention authorised is limited to a period of six months, except where this period is extended by the chief medical officer of the institution. Such an extension cannot be for more than six months at a time and the total period of detention of a temporary patient cannot exceed two years.

Detained persons—their rights, etc.[3]
When the Inspector of Mental Hospitals visits a mental hospital he is required to give special attention to the state of mind of any detained person the propriety of whose detention he doubts or has been requested by the patient or another person to investigate. If he thinks that the patient's condition calls for it,

[2] Sections 158 to 161 and 184 to 189 of 1945 Act (as amended and adapted) and Part V of the Mental Treatment Regulations, 1961.
[3] Sections 203 to 229 of 1945 Act.

the case is further examined and the Minister may then direct the patient's discharge.

Detained persons may be allowed to be absent on trial for periods up to ninety days or on parole for periods up to forty-eight hours. They may also be boarded-out indefinitely in private dwellings, while remaining under surveillance by the medical staff of the mental hospital.

When a patient detained under a reception order recovers, his relatives are told and he is discharged. He cannot then be taken back into detention in a hospital except by the making of a fresh reception order.

There are several other safeguards contained in the Mental Treatment Acts against wrongful detention of patients. The principal ones are:

(a) Every patient has a right to have a letter forwarded, un-opened, to the Minister, the President of the High Court, the Registrar of Wards of Court, the health board, or the Inspector of Mental Hospitals. The Minister may arrange for an examination of a patient by the Inspector of Mental Hospitals and may direct his discharge where justified. The President of the High Court may require the Inspector to visit and examine any patient detained as a person of unsound mind and report to him.

(b) Any person may apply to the Minister for an order for the examination, by two medical practitioners, of a patient detained and the Minister may, if he thinks fit, on consideration of their report, direct the discharge of the patient.

(c) The Act specifically requires that a patient who has recovered must be discharged.

(d) Penalties are imposed by the Act for detention otherwise than in accordance with the provisions of the Act.

(e) Any relative or friend of a person detained may apply for the discharge of a patient and, if the medical officer of the institution certifies that the patient is dangerous or otherwise unfit for discharge, an appeal lies to the Minister.

Voluntary patients[4]

A patient may, without the recommendation of a medical prac-

---

[4]Sections 190 to 196 of 1945 Act (as amended and adapted).

titioner, apply to be admitted for treatment in a mental hospital as a voluntary patient. A person admitted in this way may leave the hospital at any time on giving three days' notice. Where a person is under sixteen years of age, application for admission must be made by his parent or guardian, and must be accompanied by a recommendation from a registered medical practitioner.

Special provisions on detention of mental patients[5]
Because of the nature of their illness, there are a number of special restrictions in connection with the keeping and treatment of mental patients. To keep a person of unsound mind in an unregistered institution is an offence. Concealment of a patient in a mental hospital, assisting such a patient to escape and ill-treatment or neglect of a patient all carry heavy penalties and the use of mechanical means of restraining patients is subject to stringent regulation. The Regulations require that 'patients in a mental institution shall be treated with all gentleness compatible with their condition, and restraint, when necessary, shall be as moderate, both in extent and duration, as is consistent with the safety and advantage of the patients'. Dietaries, bathing, visiting hours and correspondence are also among the subjects covered by the Regulations.[6]

The Inspector of Mental Hospitals
The Minister for Health is required to appoint a registered medical practitioner as Inspector of Mental Hospitals.[7] The Inspector has wide duties and powers in relation to the inspection of mental hospitals and the patients in them.[8] He regularly visits each mental institution on a general inspection and may, at any time of the day or night, enter and inspect any such institution and examine any patient. All reasonable facilities for his inspections must be afforded to him. His annual reports, which he makes to the Minister, are published.[9]

Criminal lunatics
A criminal lunatic may be described as any person who, while

[5]Various provisions of Part XIX of 1945 Act (as amended and adapted).
[6]Articles 18 to 32 of Mental Treatment (Regulations) Order, 1946.
[7]Section 12 of 1945 Act.
[8]Sections 235 to 248 of 1945 Act.
[9]They are available from the Stationery Office.

in custody, has been certified to be insane in any of the following circumstances:

  (a) while on remand or awaiting trial;
  (b) while undergoing sentence either in local or convict prison;
  (c) while awaiting the pleasure of the Government, having been found insane by a jury on arraignment; or
  (d) while awaiting the pleasure of the Government, having been found 'guilty but insane' by a jury.

Criminal lunatics are confined either in the Central Mental Hospital, Dundrum[10] or in the district mental hospitals, on the order of the Minister for Justice. The case defined at (a) must be sent to the district mental hospital serving the area where the person is in custody, while cases at (b) undergoing sentence in a convict prison must be sent to Dundrum when certified insane. The Minister for Justice has discretion to send other cases either to the district mental hospital or to Dundrum.

---

[10]This hospital (originally called the Central Criminal Lunatic Asylum) is governed by the Central Criminal Lunatic Asylum (Ireland) Act, 1845, and section 44 of the Health Act, 1970.

APPENDIX I

Registration of Births, Deaths and Marriages:
Vital Statistics

Registration

Two Acts passed in 1863[1] saw the commencement of the present comprehensive system for the registration of births, deaths and marriages. Until then there was no civil registration of births or deaths in Ireland and the registration of marriages did not extend to marriages in Catholic Churches (which were much more numerous than other forms of marriage). The system of registration established in 1863 has not been altered in any major respect up to the present. It is based on local registrars under the supervision of superintendent registrars, who, in turn, are under an tArd-Chláraitheóir (the Registrar-General).[2]

Registration of births
The local registrar has the duty of registering all births which take place in his district. He keeps the register in local premises and the informant attends there to give the information necessary for registration and to sign the register. The duty of doing this rests primarily on the parents and, in their default, on the occupier of the house where the child was born, on each person present at the birth and on the person in charge of the child.[3] In practice, the informants for the registration of most births are the authorities of the maternity hospitals. The information recorded is the date and place of the birth, the name and sex of the child, the name, surname and dwelling-place of the father, the name, surname and maiden surname of the mother and the rank or profession of the father.

Each quarter, the registrar sends to the superintendent

---

[1] These, and the later amending Registration Acts, are listed in Appendix J.
[2] The Registrar-General is an autonomous officer, but the exercise of some of his functions is subject to control by the Minister for Health.
[3] Section 1 of the Births and Deaths Registration Act (Ireland), 1880.

registrar[4] a copy of the entries made by him in his register. The superintendent checks and certifies these and sends them to Oifig an tArd-Chláraitheóra. The local registrar keeps the register-book until it is filled, when he sends it to the superintendent registrar for retention. The copies of the entries in the local registers which are received in Oifig an tArd-Chláraitheóra (the General Register Office) are indexed and micro-filmed.

Birth certificates
Birth certificates are issued by Oifig an tArd-Chláraitheóra, the superintendent registrars and the local registrars. The last-named can only issue certificates of comparatively recent registrations as their register books when completed are sent to the superintendent registrar. Any member of the public is entitled, on paying a fee, to a certified copy of an entry in a register.

Two forms of certificate are issued, the full certificate, which is a true copy of the entry and the short certificate, on which is shown only the name, surname, sex and date of birth of the person and the district of registration.[5] The fee for the full certificate is 30p and that for the short certificate is $7\frac{1}{2}$p. In each case there is a search fee of $17\frac{1}{2}$p if, as is most common, the register or index must be searched to identify the entry, so that the usual full cost is $47\frac{1}{2}$p for a full certificate and 25p for a short one.[6] Of the certificates issued from Oifig an tArd-Chláraitheóra, over 50 per cent are now in the short form.

Certificates required for some special purposes, such as to accompany applications for children's allowances and other Social Welfare benefits, are obtainable from local registrars and superintendent registrars at a special fee of 5p.

---

[4]The Clerk of the Local Poor Law Union was named by section 22 of the Registration of Births and Deaths (Ireland) Acts, 1863, as superintendent registrar. His successor in the public assistance administration was later designated to act as superintendent. Under section 10 of the Vital Statistics and Births, Deaths and Marriages Registration Act, 1952, the public assistance authority took over the functions of the superintendent registrar whenever a vacancy occurred. The health boards have now replaced the public assistance authorities as superintendent registrars (section 6 of the Health Act, 1970) and discharge this function through nominated officers.
[5]The short form was introduced by the Short Birth Certificate Regulations, 1953.
[6]The fee for the full certificate and the search fee are fixed by articles 7 and 8 of the Registration of Births, Deaths and Marriages (Alteration of Fees and Allowances) Regulations, 1965: that for the short certificate is fixed by the Short Birth Certificate Regulations, 1953.

Registration of deaths and issue of death certificates
The duty of registering all deaths which take place in his district also falls on the local registrar. In the case of a death taking place in a house, the obligation to inform the registrar rests, in the order of priority shown, on:

(a) the nearest relatives of the deceased present at his death or in attendance during his last illness,
(b) every other relative living or being in the same district as the deceased,
(c) each person present at the death,
(d) the occupier of the house or hospital where the death took place,
(e) each other inmate of the house,
(f) the person causing the body to be buried.

Rather similar priorities of obligation to register apply where a death occurs or where a dead body is found elsewhere than in a house.[7] The items registered are the date and place of the death, the name, surname, sex, conjugal condition, age and occupation of the deceased and the cause of death. The cause of death is usually certified by the medical practitioner who attended the deceased in his last illness. Where a post mortem or an inquest has been held, a coroner's certificate as to the cause is sent to the registrar. The death registers are checked, copied and indexed in the same way as the registers of births and the procedure and charges for certificates issued by the registrars are similar. The reduced fee for death certificates required for special purposes, such as Social Welfare benefits, is $7\frac{1}{2}$p.

Registration of marriages
By an Act passed in 1844,[8] the registration of marriages, other than those in Catholic Churches, was initiated through specially-appointed local registrars of marriages. At the same time the office of the Registrar-General of Marriages was established. Copies of the local registers were sent to this office and central recording of these marriages commenced. Registration through different channels of Catholic marriages was in-

[7] Sections 10 and 11 of Births and Deaths Registration Act, (Ireland), 1880.
[8] Marriages (Ireland) Act, 1844.

troduced in 1863, when it was arranged that a certificate signed by the priest, the parties to the marriage and the witnesses, would be sent to the registrar of births and deaths. He was required to keep a register of such marriages and subsequent steps as respects checking, copying, indexing and the issue of certificates were prescribed as for registers of births and deaths. These parallel procedures for registration of marriages continue today. The form of the marriage register is, however, the same in each case, the particulars required being the date of the marriage and, for each of the contracting parties, the name and surname, date of birth, previous marital condition, occupation, place of residence before and after marriage, name and surname of father and name and maiden surname of mother.[9]

Vital Statistics

Statistics of births, deaths and marriages
The basic vital statistics are those of births, deaths and marriages. From the establishment of his office, the Registrar-General had the duty of publishing annual abstracts of these statistics. These Reports of the Registrar-General are the sources of most of the vital statistics for the period up to 1952, when the Registrar-General was relieved of this duty.[10] Under an Act passed in that year, the Minister for Health was given power to compile and publish vital statistics and to do this, if he wished, through the agency of other Government Offices.[11] This placed on a formal basis an arrangement under which the statistical work which stemmed from the registration system was done by the Central Statistics Office.

The Vital Statistics Regulations, 1954
From 1 January 1955, an improved system was introduced for collecting statistics of births and deaths. Before then only the information required to be given for registering a birth or death was available to the statistical service. This was not sufficient to allow for the production of some desirable statistical tables and indices. In relation to births, for example, it was not

[9]The form now in use is prescribed in the Marriages (Amendment of Form of Register and Certificates) Regulations, 1956.
[10]Section 11 of Vital Statistics and Births, Deaths and Marriages Registration Act, 1952.
[11]Section 2 of the same Act.

known what number of previous children there were in the family or what the mother's age was—both important factors in calculating fertility rates and making population forecasts.

Under the new system which started in 1955, statistical forms were introduced for completion by the informant at the registration of a birth or death. These forms provide for the items already required for registration and information to be used for the compilation of statistics. The complete list of relevant items on the birth form is:

(a)　date and place of birth of the child;
(b)　sex of the child;
(c)　name and dwelling place of the father;
(d)　occupation of the father;
(e)　date of birth of the mother;
(f)　dwelling place of the mother before the birth;
(g)　year of present marriage of the mother;
(h)　number of children of the mother by her present or any previous husband—
　　　(i)　born alive and still living,
　　　(ii)　born alive, but dead at the time the particulars are furnished.[12]

The headings on the form for deaths are:

(a)　date and place of death;
(b)　name and home address of deceased person;
(c)　sex of deceased person;
(d)　whether the deceased person was married, widowed or single;
(e)　age of the deceased person (in hours if under one day, in completed days if under one month, in completed months if under one year and otherwise in completed years);
(f)　the occupation of the deceased person, or where the deceased person was a child, the occupation of the parent or guardian;
(g)　if the deceased person was a married or widowed

[12]Article 3 of the Vital Statistics Regulations, 1954, as amended by the Vital Statistics (Amendment) Regulations, 1957.

female, the occupation of her husband.[13]

The registrar verifies that the forms are properly completed and sends them to the Central Statistics Office.

Foetal deaths
The collection of information on foetal deaths is a feature of the vital statistics in most modern states. Comprehensive, systematic collection of these statistics commenced in Ireland from 1 January 1957.[14] When foetal death occurs after the twenty-eighth week of pregnancy, the medical practitioner or midwife (or medical student or pupil midwife) is required to send information about it to the local medical officer. Forms for this purpose are provided by the health board. The headings under which information is given on the form are:

(a)   date and place of the confinement;
(b)   estimated period of gestation;
(c)   sex of the foetus;
(d)   putative cause of the foetal death;
(e)   name and normal dwelling place of mother;
(f)   date of birth of the mother;
(g)   years of present marriage of the mother;
(h)   number of previous children of the mother (by her present or any previous husband)—
      (i) still living,
      (ii) born alive but now dead;
(i)   number of previous foetal deaths (if any) as respects the mother.

The form is in two parts: that with the name and address of the mother is kept by the medical officer and he sends the remainder of the form to the Central Statistics Officer. Statistics of foetal deaths are included in the Reports on Vital Statistics.

[13]Article 4 of the Vital Statistics Regulations, 1954.
[14]Under the Vital Statistics (Foetal Deaths) Regulations, 1956, of which the succeeding sentences above are a summary.

Table of Acts, Regulations and General Orders

List of Contents

Abbreviations: am. = amended; rep. = repealed; rev. = revoked. References to amending Acts and regulations are to those in the same series, unless otherwise stated

Titles of Acts, Regulations and Orders	Provisions repealed, revoked or amended
Establishment and Functions of Department of Health:	
Ministers and Secretaries (Amendment) Act, 1946 (No. 38).	
Health (Transfer of Departmental Administration and Ministerial Functions) Order, 1947 (S.R. & O. 58).	Para. 5 of Second Schedule adapted by Health Act, 1947 (Adaptation) Order, 1948 (S.I. 101).
Agriculture and Health (Transfer of Departmental Administration and Ministerial Functions) Order, 1947 (S.R. & O. 417).	
Health (Transfer of Departmental Administration and Ministerial Functions) Order, 1949 (S.I. 256).	
Health (Transfer of Departmental Administration and Ministerial Functions) Order, 1950 (S.I. 138).	
Health (Transfer of Departmental Administration and Ministerial Functions) Order, 1958 (S.I. 202).	
General Health Legislation:	
Venereal Diseases Act, 1917 (7 & 8 Geo. V. c. 21).	
Rats and Mice (Destruction) Act, 1919 (9 & 10 Geo. V. c. 72).	Ss. 2 and 9 rep. in Part by Local Government (Repeal of Enactments) Act, 1950; S. 8 am. by S. 106 of Health Act, 1947; S. 11 extended by S. 79 of Health Act, 1970.
Registration of Maternity Homes Act, 1934 (No. 14).	S. 1 adapted by Health Act, 1970 (Adaptation) Regulations, 1971.

TABLE OF ACTS, REGULATIONS AND GENERAL ORDERS

Titles of Acts, Regulations and Orders	Provisions repealed, revoked or amended
Tuberculosis (Establishment of Sanatoria) Act, 1945 (No. 4).	S. 6 am. (S. 19 of Health Act, 1947 and S. 70 of Health Act, 1953); new S. 18 added by S. 70 of Health Act, 1953.
Mental Treatment Act, 1945 (No. 19).	*Repeals:* Ss. 3 (in part), 5, 14, 18-29, 31, 34-39, 40-62, 83, 84, 95-98, 100-106, 197-202, 208(4), 216(2), 223, 226, 227, 232-234, 238, 248(4) and 248(5).
	Amendments: A considerable number of amendments were effected by the 1961 Act and several adaptations to bring the Act into conformity with the Health Act, 1970 were made by the Mental Treatment Acts (Adaptation) Regulations, 1971.
Health Act, 1947 (No. 28).	*Repeals:* Parts II, III and VII, Ss. 41, 44 (subsections (4), (7) and (8)), 55, 67, 73, 101, 102 and 104 (subsection (7) of S. 44 by Health Services (Financial Provisions) Act, 1947—rest by Health Acts, 1953 and 1970).
	Amendments: Ss. 31, 38, 44, 48, Part V, 65, 66, 98, 193, 104 and 195 (Part IV and S. 66 of 1953 Act). See S. 4 of 1953 Act re offences under Parts V, VIII or IX. S. 65 am. by Misuse of Drugs Act, 1977.
	Adaptations: Ss. 59(a) (iii), 91(c), 91(e), 93(2), 94(2) and 94(4) adapted by Health Act, 1970 (Adaptation) Regulations, 1971.
Health Act, 1953 (No. 26).	*Repeals:* Parts II and III, Ss. 45 to 53 and 71 by 1970 Act.
	Adaptations: Ss. 62, 64(2) and 68(3) adapted by Health Act, 1970 (Adaptation) Regulations, 1971.

TABLE OF ACTS, REGULATIONS AND GENERAL ORDERS

Titles of Acts, Regulations and Orders	Provisions repealed, revoked or amended
Voluntary Health Insurance Act, 1957 (No. 1).	
Health Authorities Act, 1960 (No. 9).	*Repeals:* the whole Act (except Ss. 15(8), 15(9), 24 and the Fourth Schedule) by the Health Act, 1970. *Adaptations:* S. 15(8) (e) by Health Act, 1970 (Adaptation) Regulations, 1971; S. 24 by Health Act, 1970 (Adaptation) Regulations, 1975.
Health (Fluoridation of Water Supplies) Act, 1960 (No. 46).	
Mental Treatment Act, 1961 (No. 7).	Several adaptations were effected by the Mental Treatment Acts (Adaptation) Order, 1971.
Health (Corporate Bodies) Act, 1961 (No. 27).	*Adaptation:* S. 7(2) by Health Act, 1970 (Adaptation) Regulations, 1971.
Health (Homes for Incapacitated Persons) Act, 1964 (No. 8).	
Health Act, 1970 (No. 1).	
International Health Bodies (Corporate Status) Act, 1971 (No. 1).	
Health Contributions Act, 1971 (No. 21).	
Health Contributions (Amendment) Act, 1978 (No. 6).	
Tobacco Products (Control of Advertising, Sponsorship and Sales Promotion) Act, 1978 (No. 27).	

TABLE OF ACTS, REGULATIONS AND GENERAL ORDERS

Titles of Acts, Regulations and Orders	Provisions repealed, revoked or amended
General Regulations and Orders:	
Health Act, 1970 (Commencement) Order, 1970 (S.I. 47).	
Health Boards Regulations, 1970 (S.I. 170).	Art. 10 am. by Health (Local Committee) Regulations, 1977.
Health Act, 1970 (Commencement) Order, 1971 (S.I. 90).	
Health Services Regulations, 1971 (S.I. 105).	Art. 6 am. by Health Services Regulations, 1974.
	Art. 8 rev. by Health Services (Amendment) Regulations, 1971.
Health Act, 1970 (Adaptation) Regulations, 1971 (S.I. 106).	
Health Boards (Functions of Chief Executive Officers) Order, 1971 (S.I. 107).	
Mental Treatment Acts (Adaptation) Order, 1971 (S.I. 108).	
Health Officers (Age Limit) Order, 1971 (S.I. 109).	
Health (Removal of Officers and Servants) Order, 1971 (S.I. 110).	Art. 4(4) (i) am. by 1972 Regs. (S.I. 165) and by 1973 Regs. (S.I. 180).
Health Authorities (Dissolution) Order, 1971 (S.I. 117).	
Joint Health Boards (Dissolution) Order, 1971 (S.I. 118).	
Health Act, 1970 (Commencement) (No. 2.) Order, 1971 (S.I. 272).	
Health Services (Limited Eligibility) Regulations, 1971 (S.I. 276).	Art. 2 am. by 1976 Regs. (S.I. 141).

TABLE OF ACTS, REGULATIONS AND GENERAL ORDERS

Titles of Acts, Regulations and Orders	Provisions repealed, revoked or amended
Health Services (Amendment) Regulations, 1971 (S.I.277).	Arts. 6, 7 and 8 am. by 1973 Regulations (S.I. 184); Art. 8 am. by 1975 Regulations (S.I. 64).
Health Contributions Regulations, 1971 (S.I. 278).	New Art. 4 inserted by 1974 Regulations (S.I. 89); New Art. 6 inserted and Arts. 7 and 8 am. by 1974 (No. 2) Regulations (S.I. 373); Arts. 6, 7 and 8 am. by 1976 Regulations; Art. 6 am. by 1978 Regulations.
Health (Disqualification of Officers and Servants) Order, 1971 (S.I. 289).	
Health Services (Amendment) Regulations, 1971 (S.I. 239).	
Health (Local Committees) Regulations, 1972 (S.I. 31).	Art. 5 am. by 1977 Regulations; Arts. 2, 3, 4, 6, 7, 8, 10 adapted and modified by 1977 Regulations (S.I. 68).
Health Boards (Election of Members) Regulations, 1972 (S.I. 60).	
Health Act, 1970 (Adaptation) Regulations, 1972 (S.I. 65).	
Health Act, 1970 (Commencement) Order, 1972 (S.I. 87).	
Health Services Regulations, 1972 (S.I. 88).	Art. 6(1) rev. by 1975 Regulations (S.I. 181); Arts. 6(2), 6(3) and 6(4) am. by 1976 Regulations (S.I. 97).
Health (Hospital Bodies) Regulations, 1972 (S.I. 164).	
Health (Removal of Officers and Servants) (Amendment) Regulations, 1972 (S.I. 165).	

TABLE OF ACTS, REGULATIONS AND GENERAL ORDERS

Titles of Acts, Regulations and Orders	Provisions repealed, revoked or amended
General Medical Services (Payments) Board (Establishment) Order, 1972 (S.I. 184).	
Health Act, 1970 (Commencement) (No. 2) Order, 1972 (S.I. 240).	
Maternity Cash Grants Regulations, 1972 (S.I. 241).	
Health Act, 1970 (Commencement) Order, 1973 (S.I. 159).	
Health (Removal of Officers and Servants) (Amendment) Regulations, 1973 (S.I. 180).	
Health Services Regulations, 1973 (S.I. 184).	
Health Act, 1970 (Adaptation) Regulations, 1973 (S.I. 349).	
Health Contributions (Amendment) Regulations, 1974 (S.I. 89).	
Health Services Regulations, 1974 (S.I. 90).	New Art. 3 inserted by 1976 Regs; Art. 3 am. by 1978 Regs.
Health Contributions (Amendment) (No. 2) Regulations, 1974 (S.I. 373).	
Health Act, 1970 (Adaptation) Regulations, 1975 (S.I. 29).	
Health Services (Amendment) Regulations, 1975 (S.I. 64).	
Health Services Regulations, 1973 (Amendment) Regulations, 1975 (S.I. 181).	
Health Act, 1970 (Commencement) Order, 1976 (S.I. 78).	
Hospitals Commission (Dissolution) Order, 1976 (S.I. 79).	

TABLE OF ACTS, REGULATIONS AND GENERAL ORDERS

Titles of Acts, Regulations and Orders	Provisions repealed, revoked or amended
Health Contributions (Amendment) Regulations, 1976 (S.I. 80).	
Health Services Regulations, 1976 (S.I. 97).	
Health Services (Limited Eligibility) Regulations, 1976 (S.I. 141).	
Health Services (Amendment) Regulations, 1976 (S.I. 142).	
Health (Charges for in-patient services) Regulations, 1976 (S.I. 180).	
Health (Local Committees) Regulations, 1977 (S.I. 68).	
Health Contributions (Amendment) Regulations, 1978 (S.I. 98).	
Health Services Regulations, 1978 (S.I. 371).	
Infectious Diseases Regulations:	
Infectious Diseases Regulations, 1948 (S.I. 99).	Art. 3 rev. by 1967 Regs.; Art. 22 rev. by Art. 6 of 1952 Regs.; Arts. 11 and 20 am. by 1948. (Am.) Regs.; Art. 23 am. by 1958 Regs.; Art. 27 am. by 1951 Regs; Second Schedule am. by 1948 (Am.) Regs. and 1956 Regs.; Arts. 8, 9, 11, 17, 28, 29 and Second Schedule am. by 1976 Regulations.
Infectious Diseases (Aircraft) Regulations, 1948 (S.I. 136).	
Infectious Diseases (Aircraft) Regulations, 1948 (Specified Areas) Order, 1948 (S.I. 232).	
Infectious Diseases (Shipping) Regulations, 1948 (S.I. 170).	

Titles of Acts, Regulations and Orders	Provisions repealed, revoked or amended
Infectious Diseases (Amendment) Regulations, 1948 (S.I. 353).	
Prohibition from School Attendance (Notices) Regulations, 1948 (S.I. 371).	
Infectious Diseases (Amendment) Regulations, 1949 (S.I. 351).	
Infectious Diseases (Amendment) Regulations, 1951 (S.I. 318).	
Infectious Diseases (Amendment) Regulations, 1952 (S.I. 291).	
Infectious Diseases (Amendment) Regulations, 1958 (S.I. 148).	
Infectious Diseases (Certificate of Vaccination Against Smallpox) Regulations, 1966 (S.I. 23).	
Infectious Diseases (Amendment) Regulations, 1968 (S.I. 258).	
Infectious Diseases (Maintenance) Regulations, 1979 (S.I. 78).	
Food Hygiene Regulations:	
Food Hygiene Regulations, 1950 (S.I. 205).	Arts. 19, 20, 21, 22 and 23 rev. by 1971 Regs. Arts. 14, 25, 26, 40, 46 & 48 am. by 1971 Regs. Arts. 46 and 47 am. by 1952 Regs. Art. 48 am. by 1961 Regs. New articles 43A & 46 inserted by 1971 Regs.
Food Hygiene (Amendment) Regulations, 1952 (S.I. 289).	

TABLE OF ACTS, REGULATIONS AND GENERAL ORDERS

Titles of Acts, Regulations and Orders	Provisions repealed, revoked or amended
Food Hygiene Regulations, 1950 (Shellfish Controlled Areas) Order, 1951 (S.I. 16).	Paragraph (c) and (e) of Schedule revoked by 1952 Order.
Food Hygiene Regulations, 1950 (Commencement of Part IV) Order, 1951 (S.I. 270).	
Food Hygiene (Official Certificate No. 1) Order, 1952 (S.I. 94).	
Food Hygiene (Official Certificate No. 2) Order, 1952 (S.I. 150).	
Food Hygiene Regulations, 1950 (Shellfish Controlled Areas) Order, 1952 (S.I. 272).	
Food Hygiene (Official Certificate No. 3) Order, 1953 (S.I. 306).	
Food Hygiene (Official Certificate No. 4) Order, 1954 (S.I. 201).	
Food Hygiene (Official Certificate No. 5) Order, 1955 (S.I. 20).	
Food Hygiene (Official Certificate Nos. 6 & 7) Order, 1963 (S.I. 184).	
Food Hygiene Regulations, 1950 (Shellfish Controlled Area) Order, 1971 (S.I. 26).	
Food Hygiene (Amendment) Regulations, 1971 (S.I. 322).	
Food Hygiene Regulations (Shellfish Controlled Area) Order, 1977 (S.I. 113).	

TABLE OF ACTS, REGUI ʌTIONS AND GENERAL ORDERS

Titles of Acts, Regulations and Orders	Provisions repealed, revoked or amended
Food Standards Etc.:	
Public Health (Saorstát Éireann) (Preservatives in Food) Regulations, 1928 (S.R. & O. 54).	Arts. 4(1), 4(2), 5(1), 5(2), 11(1) and First & Second Schs. rev. by Public Health (Preservatives in Food Regs. 1928 & 1943) (Amd.) Regs. 1972.
	Arts. 3, 6, 7, 9, 10 and 14 adapted by Art. 4 of Health Act, 1947 (Adaptation) Order, 1951 (S.I. 15).
Food Standards (Ice-cream) Regulations, 1952 (S.I. 227).	
Health (Arsenic or Lead in Food) Regulations, 1972 (S.I. 44).	
Health (Mineral Hydrocarbons in Food) Regulations, 1972 (S.I. 45).	
Public Health (Preservatives, etc. in Food Regulations, 1928 and 1943) (Amendment) Regulations, 1972 (S.I. 46).	
Health (Solvents in Food) Regulations, 1972 (S.I. 304).	
Health (Preservatives in Food) Regulations, 1973 (S.I. 147).	
Health (Antioxidant in Food) Regulations, 1973 (S.I. 148).	
Health (Colouring Agents in Food) Regulations, 1973 (S.I. 149).	First Sch. am. by 1978 Regs.
Health (Erucic Acid in Food) Regulations, 1978 (S.I. 123).	
Health (Colouring Agents in Food) Regulations, 1978 (S.I. 140).	

Titles of Acts, Regulations and Orders	Provisions repealed, revoked or amended
Medicines:	
Pharmacopoeia Act, 1931 (No. 22).	Ss. 1, 2, 3 and 4 am. by sections 35 and 42 of Misuse of Drugs Act, 1977.
Therapeutic Substances Act, 1932 (No. 25).	
Therapeutic Substances (Advisory Committee) Rules, 1933 (S.R. & O. 106).	
Therapeutic Substances (Saorstát Éireann) Regulations, 1934 (S. R. & O. 365).	*Amendments:* Arts. 5 (1941 Regs.), 7 (1947 Regs.), 8 (1954 Regs.), 10 (1947 Regs.), 13 (1939 and 1947 Regs.), 17 (1938 Regs.), 21 (1946 and 1948 Regs.); Second Schedule (1935, 1936, 1941 and 1955 Regs.); Sixth Schedule added by 1939 Regs.; Seventh Schedule added by 1947 Regs.
Therapeutic Substances (Saorstát Éireann) (Amendment) Regulations, 1935 (S.R. & O. 563).	Arts. 1, 2, 3, 4, 5, 6 and 9 am. by 1937 Regs.; Art. 2 am. by Art. 4 of 1941 Regs.
Therapeutic Substances (Saorstát Éireann) (Amendment) (No. 2) Regulations, 1936 (S. R. & O. 46).	
Therapeutic Substances (Amendment) Regulations, 1936 (S.R. & O. 71).	
Therapeutic Substances (Amendment) Regulations, 1937 (S.R. & O. 284).	
Therapeutic Substances (Amendment) Regulations, 1938 (S.R. & O. 21).	

Titles of Acts, Regulations and Orders	Provisions repealed, revoked or amended
Therapeutic Substances (Amendment) Regulations, 1939 (S.R. & O. 253).	
Therapeutic Substances (Amendment) Regulations, 1941 (S.R. & O. 14).	
Therapeutic Substances (Amendment) Regulations, 1946 (S.R. & O. 241).	
Therapeutic Substances (Penicillin) Order, 1946 (S.R. & O. 242).	
Therapeutic Substances (Amendment) Regulations, 1947 (S.R. & O. 345).	Art. 3 am. by 1953 Regs.
Therapeutic Substances (Amendment) Regulations, 1948 (S.I. 263).	
Therapeutic Substances (Amendment) Regulations, 1953 (S.I. 143).	
Therapeutic Substances (Fees) Regulations, 1954 (S.I. 183).	
Therapeutic Substances (Amendment) Regulations, 1954 (S.I. 198).	
Therapeutic Substances (Amendment) Regulations, 1955 (S.I. 149).	
Medical Preparations (Advertisement and Sale) Regulations, 1958 (S.I. 135).	

TABLE OF ACTS, REGULATIONS AND GENERAL ORDERS

Titles of Acts, Regulations and Orders	Provisions repealed, revoked or amended
Medical Preparations (Control of Sale) Regulations, 1966 (S.I. 261).	Arts. 4, 7 and 9 am. by 1971 Regulations; First Schedule am. by 1976 Regulations.
Medical Preparations (Control of Amphetamine) Regulations, 1969 (S.I. 244).	Sch. replaced by 1970 Regulations.
Medical Preparations (Control of Amphetamine) (Amendment) Regulations, 1970 (S.I. 137).	
Medical Preparations (Control of Sale) (Amendment) Regulations, 1971 (S.I. 272).	
European Communities (Proprietary Medicinal Products) Regulations, 1974 (S.I. 187).	
Medical Preparations (Licensing of Manufacture) Regulations, 1974 (S.I. 225).	
Medical Preparations (Wholesale Licences) Regulations, 1974 (S.I. 333).	
European Communities (Proprietary Medicinal Products) Regulations, 1975 (S.I. 301).	
Medical Preparations (Licensing of Manufacture) (Amendment) Regulations, 1975 (S.I. 302).	
Medical Preparations (Control of Sale) (Amendment) Regulations, 1976 (S.I. 82).	

TABLE OF ACTS, REGULATIONS AND GENERAL ORDERS

Titles of Acts, Regulations and Orders	Provisions repealed, revoked or, amended
Dangerous Drugs:	
Misuse of Drugs Act, 1977 (No. 12).	
Misuse of Drugs Act, 1977 (Commencement) Order, 1979 (S.I. 28).	
Misuse of Drugs (Exemption) Order, 1979 (S.I. 29).	
Misuse of Drugs (Designation) Order, 1979 (S.I. 30).	
Misuse of Drugs (Committee of Inquiry, Advisory Committees and Advisory Panels) Regulations, 1979 (S.I. 31).	
Misuse of Drugs Regulations, 1979 (S.I. 32).	

TABLE OF ACTS, REGULATIONS AND GENERAL ORDERS

Titles of Acts, Regulations and Orders	Provisions repealed, revoked or amended
Sale of Food and Drugs:*	
Sale of Food and Drugs Act, 1875 (38 & 39 Vic. c. 63).	S. 6 am. by S. 5 of 1936 Act.
Sale of Food and Drugs Amendment Act, 1879 (42 & 43 Vic. c. 30).	Ss. 3 and 4 am. by S. 3 of 1935 Act.
Margarine Act, 1887 (50 & 51 Vic. c. 29).	
Sale of Food and Drugs Act, 1899 (62 & 63 Vic. c. 51).	Ss. 9 and 11 rep. by Milk and Dairies Act, 1935; Ss. 4, 10 and 14 am. by 1935 Act.
Butter and Margarine Act, 1907 (7 Ed. 7 c. 21).	
Sale of Food and Drugs (Milk) Act, 1935 (No. 3).	Ss. 2, 7 and 8 am. by 1936 Act.
Sale of Food and Drugs (Milk) Act, 1936 (No. 44).	S. 2(4) adapted by Article 3 of Health Act, 1947 (Adaptation) Order, 1951 (S. 15).
Sale of Butter (Ireland) Regulations 1902.	
Sale of Food and Drugs (Milk Sampling Regulations, 1936 (S.R. & O. 312).	Art. 9 and Schedule am. by 1941 Regs.
Milk (Percentage of milk-fat and milk-solids) (No. 2) Regulations, 1936 (S.R. & O. 321).	
Sale of Food and Drugs (Milk Sampling) (Amendment) Regulations, 1941 (S. R. & O. 246).	

*The texts and repeals and amendments of provisions of these Acts up to 1911 and notes on case law are given in Vanston's 'Law relating to Public Health in Ireland'. Only later repeals and amendments are noted here.

TABLE OF ACTS, REGULATIONS AND GENERAL ORDERS

Titles of Acts, Regulations and Orders	Provisions repealed, revoked or amended
Poisons:	
Sections 30 & 31 of Pharmacy (Ire.) Act, 1875 (38 and 39 Vic. c. 57).	Amended by Pharmacopoeia Act, 1931.
Poisons and Pharmacy Act, 1908 (8 Ed. 7. c. 55).	Ss. 2 and 5 rep. by S. 21 of 1961 Act.
Regulations are contained in an Order of Privy Council of 29 June 1917.	
Poisons Act, 1961 (No. 12).	Ss. 4, 14 and 15 am. and new S. 15A inserted by Misuse of Drugs Act, 1977.
Poisons Act, 1961 (Paraquat) Regulations, 1975 (S.I. 146).	
Section 33(1)(c) and (2) of Misuse of Drugs Act, 1977 (No. 12).	
Miscellaneous Instruments on Services:	
Boarding-Out of Children Regulations, 1954 (S.I. 101).	
Institutional Assistance Regulations, 1954 (S.I. 103).	Art. 12 replaced by 1965 Regs.
Disabled Persons (Rehabilitation) Regulations, 1963 (S.I. 141).	
Institutional Assistance Regulations, 1965 (S.I. 177).	
Homes for Incapacitated Persons Regulations, 1966 (S.I. 44).	
International Federation of Voluntary Health Service Funds (Corporate Status) Order, 1971 (S.I. 308).	
Disabled Persons (Maintenance Allowances) Regulations, 1973 (S.I. 160).	Art. 4 am. 1979 Regs.
Disabled Persons (Maintenance Allowances) (Amendment) Regulations, 1979 (S.I. 79).	

TABLE OF ACTS, REGULATIONS AND GENERAL ORDERS

Titles of Acts, Regulations and Orders	Provisions repealed, revoked or amended
Hospitals Legislation:	
Public Hospitals Act, 1933 (No. 18).	*Repeals:* Subsections (1) to (6) of S. 20 repealed (S. 9 of 1938 Act).
	Amendments: Ss. 1 and 14(5) (by S. 43 of 1970 Act); S.I. adapted by Health Act, 1970 (Adaptation) Regulations, 1971.
Public Hospitals (Amendment) Act, 1938 (No. 21).	
Hospitals Act, 1939 (No. 4).	
Public Hospitals (Amendment) (No. 2) Act, 1939 (No. 29).	
Public Hospitals (Amendment) Act, 1940 (No. 9).	
St. Laurence's Hospital Act, 1943 (No. 3).	

Titles of Acts, Regulations and Orders	Provisions repealed, revoked or amended
Meath Hospital Act, 1951 (No. 5).	S.4(1) am. and S.4A. inserted by Health Authorities Act, 1960. S.4A adapted by Health Act, 1970 (Adaptation) Regulations, 1972.
Hospitals Federation and Amalgamation Act, 1961 (No. 21).	
Orders under Health (Corporate Bodies) Act, 1961:	
Dublin Dental Hospital (Establishment) Order, 1963 (S.I. 129).	Art. 4 am. by 1966 Order; Arts. 6 and 20 am. by 1964 Order; new Article 24 inserted by 1964 Order; Arts. 16 and 18 am. by 1975 Order; new Art. 25 inserted by 1975 Order.
Dublin Dental Hospital (Establishment) Order, 1963 (Amendment) Order, 1964 (S.I. 260).	
Hospitals Sterile Supplies Board (Establishment) Order, 1965 (S.I. 1).	Arts. 4, 5 and 17 am. by Amendment Order, 1965.
The Blood Transfusion Service Board (Establishment) Order, 1965 (S.I. 78).	
The Medico-Social Research Board (Establishment) Order, 1965 (S.I. 80).	Art. 5 am. by Amendment Order, 1974.
Hospitals Sterile Supplies Board (Establishment) Order, 1965 (Amendment) Order, 1965 (S.I. 157).	

TABLE OF ACTS, REGULATIONS AND GENERAL ORDERS

Titles of Acts, Regulations and Orders	Provisions repealed, revoked or amended
Dublin Dental Hospital (Establishment) Order, 1963 (Amendment) Order, 1966 (S.I. 3).	
The Cork Hospitals Board (Establishment) Order, 1966 (S.I. 133).	Art. 4 am. by 1967 Order; Arts. 4, 5, 6, 8, 21 and 22 am. by 1971 Order; Art. 5 am. by 1973 Order.
The National Drugs Advisory Board (Establishment) Order, 1966 (S.I. 163).	Art. 4 am. by 1974 Amendment Order.
The Cork Hospitals Board (Establishment) Order, 1966 (Amendment) Order, 1967 (S.I. 211).	
The National Rehabilitation Board (Establishment) Order, 1967 (S.I. 300).	
James Connolly Memorial Hospital Board (Establishment) Order, 1971 (S.I. 97).	
The Cork Hospitals Board (Establishment) Order, 1966 (Amendment) Order, 1971 (S.I. 104).	
St. James's Hospital Board (Establishment) Order, 1971 (S.I. 187).	
Health (Hospital Bodies) Regulations, 1972 (S.I. 164).	Art. 4 am. by 1978 Amendment Regs.
The Cork Hospitals Board (Establishment) Order, 1966 (Amendment) Order, 1973 (S.I. 8).	

TABLE OF ACTS, REGULATIONS AND GENERAL ORDERS

Titles of Acts, Regulations and Orders	Provisions repealed, revoked or amended
Hospital Bodies Administrative Bureau (Establishment) Order, 1973 (S.I. 53).	
The Medico-Social Research Board (Establishment) Order, 1965 (Amendment) Order, 1974 (S.I. 169).	
National Drugs Advisory Board (Establishment) Order, 1966 (Amendment) Order, 1974.	
The Health Education Bureau (Establishment) Order, 1975 (S.I. 22).	
Dublin Dental Hospital (Establishment) Order, 1963 (Amendment) Order, 1975 (S.I. 88).	
James Connolly Memorial Hospital Board (Establishment) Order, 1971 (Amendment) Order, 1977 (S.I. 135).	
Beaumont Hospital Board (Establishment) Order, 1977 (S.I. 255).	
Cork Voluntary Hospitals Board (Establishment) Order, 1977 (S.I. 290).	
Health (Hospital Bodies) Regulations, 1972 (Amendment) Regulations, 1978 (S.I. 338).	
Regulation of Professions *Medical Practitioners:*	
Medical Practitioners Act, 1978 (No. 4).	

TABLE OF ACTS, REGULATIONS AND GENERAL ORDERS

Titles of Acts, Regulations and Orders	Provisions repealed, revoked or amended
Medical Practitioners Act, 1978 (Commencement) Order, 1978 (S.I. 196).	
The Medical Council (Election of Members) Regulations, 1978 (S.I. 197).	
Dentists:	
Dentists Act, 1928 (No. 25) (Regulations under this Act are made by the Dental Board, 57 Merrion Square, Dublin).	
Nurses and Midwives:	
Midwives Act, 1944 (No. 10).	*Repeals:* Part II, Ss. 23, 24, 25, 28, 38 to 42, 44, 60, 63, 64 and 65 (S. 44 by S. 8 of Nurses Act, 1961-rest by Nurses Act, 1950).
	Amendments: Ss. 26, 27, 30 to 34, 43, 44, 47, 48, 50, 51, 53, 58, 59 and 62 (all by S. 68 of Nurses Act, 1950); Definitions and S. 47 adapted by Health Act, 1970 (Adaptation) Regulations, 1971.
Nurses Act, 1950 (No. 27).	*Repeals:* Ss. 16 and 59 (by S. 8 of 1961 Act), S. 60 by Health Act, 1970.
	Amendments: Ss. 13, 24 and 60 by 1961 Act.
	Adaptations: Section 12(2)(a) by Health Act, 1970 (Adaptation) Regulations, 1973.
Nurses Act, 1961 (No. 18).	S. 4(3) rep. by Health Act, 1970.

TABLE OF ACTS, REGULATIONS AND GENERAL ORDERS

Titles of Acts, Regulations and Orders	Provisions repealed, revoked or amended
Pharmacists:	
Pharmacy Act (Ireland) 1875 (38 and 39 Vic. c. 57).	*Repeals:* S. 15 by S. 4 of 1890 Act; Ss. 16(2), 16(6), 23, 30 and 32 by 1962 Act.
	Amendments: Ss. 11 (S. 20 of 1890 Act); S. 22 (S. 4(2)(b) and 8 of 1962 Act); S. 23 (S. 9 of 1962 Act); S. 30 (S. 14(3)(c) of Poisons Act, 1961).
Pharmacy Act (Ireland) 1875 Amendment Act, 1890 (53 & 54 Vic. c. 48).	*Repeals:* Ss. 15-18 (S. 10 of 1962 Act). *Amendments:* Ss. 10, 12, 16, 17 and 19 (Ss. 6 & 7 of 1951 Act); Ss. 15 & 17 (S. 14(3)(c) of 1961 Act).
Section 7 of Poisons and Pharmacy Act, 1908.	Ss. 4 and 5 repealed by S.10(1), of 1962 Act.
Pharmacy Act, 1951 (No. 30).	
Pharmacy Act, 1962 (No. 14).	S. 2 am. by Misuse of Drugs Act, 1977 (S.34).
Section 32 of Misuse of Drugs Act, 1977 (No. 12).	

(Regulations made under these Acts are made by the Pharmaceutical Society of Ireland, 18 Shrewsbury Road, Ballsbridge, Dublin).

Opticians:

Opticians Act, 1956 (No. 17).

(The rules under this Act are made by Bord na Radharcmhastóirí, 10 Fitzwilliam Square, Dublin).

Titles of Acts, Regulations and Orders	Provisions repealed, revoked or amended
Registration of Births, etc., Vital Statistics:	
Marriages (Ireland) Act, 1844 (7 & 8 Vic. c. 81).	S. 56 rep. by 1952 Act; S. 7 am. by Marriages Act, 1936; Ss. 8, 10, 52 and 70 by 1952 Act; Ss. 19 and 20 am. by 1972 Act.
	Schedule G am. by Marriages (Amendment of Form of Register and Certificates) Regs. 1956.
	Fees under Sections 7, 14, 16, 21, 23, 27, 28, 31, 68, 69 and 70 altered by 1953, 1954 and 1965 Regs.
Marriages (Ireland) Act, 1846 (9 & 10 Vic. c. 72).	
Registration of Births and Deaths (Ireland) Act, 1863 (26 Vic. c. 11).	*Repeals:* Ss. 3 (in part), 26 (in part), 31, 32, 33, 34, 35, 36, 37, 38, 44 and 46 (all by S. 44 of 1880 Act), 49 (by 1952 Act), 51 and 55 (by 1880 Act).
	Amendments: Ss. 4, 22 and 26 (by 1952 Act), 28 (by 1936 Act), 50 and 53 (by 1952 Act), 10 (by 1972 Act).
	Fees under Ss. 50, 53 and 54 altered by 1953, 1954 and 1965 Regs.
Marriage Law (Ireland) Amendment Act, 1863 (26 Vic. c. 27).	Fees under Ss. 3 and 12 altered by 1953 and 1954 (No. 2) Regs. S. 3 am. by 1972 Act.
Registration of Marriages (Ireland) Act, 1863 (26 and 27 Vic. c. 90).	S. 16 rep. by 1952 Act. *Amendments:* Ss. 17 and 20 (by 1952 Act), 21 (by 1936 Act).
	Form A in Schedule altered by Marriages (Amendment of Forms of Register and Certificates) Regs., 1956.
	Fees under Ss. 17, 18, 19, 20 and 21 altered by 1953, 1954 and 1965 Regs.

Titles of Acts, Regulations and Orders	Provisions repealed, revoked or amended
Matrimonial Causes and Marriage Law (Ireland) Amendment Act, 1870 (33 and 34 Vic. c. 110).	*Amendments:* Ss. 34 (by Marriages Act, 1936), 35 (by 1952 Act), 33, 35, 36 and 37 (by 1972 Act).
Matrimonial Causes and Marriage Law (Ireland) Amendment Act, 1871 (34 and 35 Vic. c. 49).	Form in Schedule A altered by Marriages (Amendment of Form of Register and Certificates) Regs., 1956.
Marriage Law (Ireland) Amendment Act, 1873 (36 Vic. c. 16).	
Births and Deaths Registration Act (Ireland), 1880 (43 and 44 Vic. c. 13).	Ss. 8, 21 and 22 and Form A in First Schedule am. by Ss. 5 and 10 of 1952 Act; S. 28 am. by S. 6 of Births, Deaths and Marriages Registration Act, 1972. Fees under Ss. 23, 24 and 25 and Second Schedule altered by 1953, 1954 and 1965 Regs.
Registration of Births and Deaths Act, 1936 (No. 34).	Allowances in S. 3 altered by Art. 3 of 1954 (No. 3) Regs. and by Art. 3 of 1965 Regs.
Registration of Marriages Act, 1936 (No. 35).	Allowance in S. 2 altered by Art. 4 of 1954 (No. 3) Regs. and by Art. 4 of 1965 Regs.
Marriages Act, 1936 (No. 47).	
Vital Statistics and Births, Deaths and Marriages Registration Act, 1952 (No. 8).	S. 2 am. by S. 7 of Births, Deaths and Marriages Registration Act, 1972.
Section 22 of Adoption Act, 1952 (No. 25).	am. by S. 7 of Adoption Act, 1964 (No. 2) and by S. 10 of Adoption Act, 1974 (No. 24).
Coroners Act, 1962 (No. 9). Births, Deaths and Marriages Registration Act, 1972 (No. 25).	

TABLE OF ACTS, REGULATIONS AND GENERAL ORDERS

Titles of Acts, Regulations and Orders	Provisions repealed, revoked or amended
Marriages Act, 1972 (No. 30).	
Social Welfare (Certificates of Births, Marriages and Deaths) Regulations, 1952 (S. I. 384).	
Oifig an Ard-Chlaraitheora (Hours of Business) Regulations, 1953 (S.I. 60).	
Births, Deaths and Marriages (Fees for Certificates) Regulations, 1953 (S.I. 61).	
Registration of Births, Deaths and Marriages (Alteration of Fees) Regulations, 1953 (S.I. 214).	Art. 3 am. by 1954 and 1965 Regs.
Short Birth Certificate Regulations, 1953 (S.I. 215).	
Registration of Births, Deaths and Marriages (Alteration of Fees) Regulations, 1954 (S.I. 144).	
Registration of Births, Deaths and Marriages (Alteration of Fees) (No. 2) Regulations, 1954 (S.I. 223).	
Registration of Births, Deaths and Marriages (Alteration of Fees) (No. 3) Regulations, 1954 (S.I. 279).	
Legitimacy Act (Alteration of Registration Fee) Regulations, 1954 (S.I. 224).	
Vital Statistics Regulations, 1954 (S.I. 280).	Art. 3 am. by 1957 Regs.
Marriages (Amendment of Form of Register and Certificates) Regulations, 1956 (S.I. 47).	

TABLE OF ACTS, REGULATIONS AND GENERAL ORDERS

Titles of Acts, Regulations and Orders	Provisions repealed, revoked or, amended
Factories Act, 1955 (Birth Certificates) Regulations, 1956 (S.I. 248).	
Vital Statistics (Foetal Deaths) Regulations, 1956 (S.I. 302).	
Vital Statistics (Amendment) Regulations, 1957 (S.I. 261).	
Registration of Births, Deaths and Marriages (Alteration of Fees and Allowances) Regulations, 1965 (S.I. 24).	

BIBLIOGRAPHY OF IRISH PUBLICATIONS

Official Publications (published by the Stationery Office)

White Paper: Outline of Proposals for the Improvement of the
Health Services, 1947 (P. No. 8400)

White Paper: Reconstruction and Improvement of County
Homes, 1951 (Pr. 756)

White Paper: Proposals for Improved and Extended Health
Services, 1952 (Pr. 1333)

Report on the Incidence of Dental Caries in School Children,
1965 (Pr. 8125)

Report of Commission of Enquiry on Mental Handicap, 1965
(Pr. 8234)

Report of Commission of Enquiry on Mental Illness, 1966
(Pr. 9181)

White Paper: The Health Services and their Further Development, 1966 (Pr. 8653)

Commission on Higher Education 1960-67—Presentation and
Summary of Report, 1967 (Pr. 9326)

The Child Health Services—Report of a Study Group, 1967
(Pr. 171)

Commission on Higher Education 1960-67—Report (Volume I)
(Pr. 9389)

Outline of the Future Hospital System—Report of the Consultative Council on the General Hospital Services
(Prl. 154)

The Care of the Aged—Report of the Interdepartmental Committee, 1968 (Prl. 777)

Report of Public Services Organisation Review Group, 1966—
1969 (Prl. 792)

Reformatory and Industrial Schools Systems Report, 1970
(Prl. 1342)

White Paper: Local Government Reorganisation, 1971 (Prl.
1572)

Report of Food Hygiene Advisory Committee on Education and
Training, 1971 (Prl. 1773)

269

Report of Working Party on Drug Abuse, 1971 (Prl. 1774)

Psychiatric Nursing Services of Health Boards—Report of Working Party, 1973 (Prl. 3043)

Restructuring the Department of Health—The Separation of Policy and Execution, 1974 (Prl. 3445)

Report of the Committee on Drug Education, 1974

The General Practitioner in Ireland—Report of the Consultative Council on General Medical Practice, 1974 (Prl. 3621)

Training and Employing the Handicapped—Report of a Working Party established by the Minister for Health, 1975 (Prl. 4302)

Survey of Workload of Public Health Nurses—Report of Working Group appointed by the Minister for Health, 1975 (Prl. 4315)

Task Force on Child Care Services—Interim Report, 1975 (Prl. 4915)

Report of the Working Party on Prescribing and Dispensing in the General Medical Services, 1976 (Prl. 5531)

Report of the Committee on Non-Accidental Injury to Children, 1976 (Prl. 5538)

Statistical Information relevant to the Health Services (editions for 1976, 1977, 1978)

Some Major Issues in Health Policy—Report of National Economic and Social Council, Report No. 29, 1977 (Prl. 5821)

Universality and Selectivity: Strategies in Social Policy—Report of National Economic and Social Council, Report No. 36, 1978 (Prl. 6416)

Universality and Selectivity: Social Services in Ireland—Report of National Economic and Social Council, Report No. 38, 1978 (Prl. 6802)

Annual Reports of the National Health Council

Other Publications

F. B. Chubb The Government: An Introduction to the Cabinet system in Ireland Second Edition (Institute of Public Administration Dublin 1968)

Seamus O Cinneide A Law for the Poor—A Study of Home Assistance in Ireland (Institute of Public Administration Dublin 1970)

J. Collins Local Government Third Edition ed D. Roche (Institute of Public Administration Dublin 1975)

S. Dooney The Irish Civil Service (Institute of Public Administration Dublin 1964)

D. Farley Social Insurance and Social Assistance in Ireland (Institute of Public Administration Dublin 1964)

Dr G. Fitzgerald State-Sponsored Bodies (Institute of Public Administration Dublin 1968)

P. R. Kaim-Caudle Social Security in Ireland and Western Europe (Economic and Social Research Institute Dublin 1964)

P. R. Kaim-Caudle Dental Services in Ireland (Economic and Social Research Institute Dublin 1969)

P. R. Kaim-Caudle Ophthalmic Services in Ireland (Economic and Social Research Institute Dublin 1970)

P. R. Kaim-Caudle Pharmaceutical Services in Ireland (Economic and Social Research Institute Dublin 1970)

D. E. Leon Advisory Bodies in Irish Government (Institute of Public Administration Dublin 1963)

J. D. O'Donnell How Ireland is Governed Third Edition (Institute of Public Administration Dublin 1979)

J. McGowan Smyth The Houses of the Oireachtas Third Edition (Institute of Public Administration Dublin 1964)

Reports of Comhairle na nOspidéal[1]

Annual Report of the General Medical Services (Payments) Board

Annual Report of the Medical Research Council[1]

Annual Report of the Medico-Social Research Board[1]

Annual Report of the National Drugs Advisory Board[1]

Annual Report of the Voluntary Health Insurance Board[1]

---

[1]These Reports are published by the bodies concerned; their addresses are listed in Appendix A.

INDEX